Loving Yoga
Enjoy Your Pra...
by Mis...

CHAPTER 1. INWARD SPIRAL *2*

CHAPTER 2. SANCTUARY *12*

CHAPTER 3. OPENING SALUTATION / MEDITATION *14*

CHAPTER 4. PRANAYAMAS *17*

CHAPTER 5. BASIC MEDITATION *36*

CHAPTER 6. GETTING PHYSICAL *45*

CHAPTER 7. PARTNERED POSTURES *65*

CHAPTER 8. THE CHAKRAS *82*

CHAPTER 9. LIFE IN BALANCE *108*

CHAPTER 10. SEX AS GOOD MEDICINE *136*

CHAPTER 11. THE ART OF AFTER *139*

©2024 1 to 1 Publishers
12439 Mafnolia Blvd., Suite 100
Valley Village, CA 91607
818-508-1296

www.1to1publishers.com

All rights reserved. No part of this book may be reproduced or transmitted in any form or by any means, electronic or mechanical, including photocopying, recording, or introduced into any information storage and retrieval system, without permission in writing from the publisher.

Disclaimer: Contact your doctor before beginning any yoga program. The advice presented in this book is in no way intended as a substitute for medical consultation, and the publisher disclaims any liability from, and in connection with, this program. If at any point while moving into and out of the poses described in this book you begin to feel faint, dizzy, or have physical discomfort, you should stop immediately and consult a physician.

Chapter 1: Inward Spiral - Self Care

All of life is full of relationship: parent/child, husband/wife, friend/lover, employer/employee, teacher/student, client/provider and so on. This means that most of us spend a lot of our time and energy in a giving role. So before you do another thing... stop, drop, and remember that a healthy sense of well-being and balance is rooted first in a positive relationship with yourself.

The bottom line is that it is important to spend some time that is for you and you alone. You cannot get it all from your partner.

Take responsibility for your own well-being. All guilty pleasures are encouraged if it helps you to make room in your life for pause - a dynamic pause that declares a shift of focus from outside to inside... a pause in which we offer to Self the energies usually consumed by others. A pause that retrieves what has been lost, calling home fragments of your soul from past and future, from daydream and anxiety... a suspended moment in which we receive the abundance of our own life force by directing it with will and awareness to extend into the deeper peace of the body. Here we find the simple pleasure of truly coming home.

As your focus returns to self, you become receptive to the abundant support of your innate life force. Your deep awareness of *I Am* infuses your being with vitality as your energies turn toward restoring balance and replenishing reservoirs depleted by constant giving.

In giving yourself back to yourself you will know a wholeness that transcends need. Without need, you can reach out to your partner from the fullness of your being - a wonderful place of equilibrium that allows a most satisfying exchange to take place. The energy gained in these moments opens the heart to freely give and freely receive.

The following are a few short trails that lead to instant bliss...well, almost.

A ROMANTIC BATH

A luxurious bath or a refreshing shower makes a wonderful transition from ordinary activities to a highly special occasion. Fill the room with candlelight. Woo yourself.

Simple Soak:
Try adding drops of essential oils like Rose, Ylang Ylang, or Jasmine to your tub to alleviate stress. Add the soothing notes of Sandalwood, Vanilla or Patchouli oil for balance. Just a few drops of each will do it. Cover your face with a warm washcloth and relax.

Superb Relaxing Bath:
This soak can arouse sensuality while inviting a lucid mind into your relaxed body... a powerful combination that produces pleasure.
- 1 ounce ginger root, grated and tied up in a loose cheesecloth bag
- Two cups Epsom salts - swish water around until the salts dissolve
- A few drops of your favorite essential oils
- A handful of flower petals - Rose, Chamomile, or Lavender are good choices and easy to find dried or fresh. Look for whatever is in season and in your environment.
- Get in and soak for at least 15 minutes, while all the emotional and physical residues accumulated in a day fall away. When you get out, dry yourself briskly with your towel to slough off dead skin and leave yourself positively radiant.

SELF MASSAGE

Preferably, situate in a sundrenched location for extra melting goodness. Use pure natural oils like Sesame, Coconut, or Almond.
- Move from your feet upwards to the tops of your thighs.
- Massage your fingers and hands.
- Drift up your arms and across your chest, one arm at a time.
- Stroke your belly and give yourself some love.
- Touch your erogenous zones - breasts, inner thighs, ears and lips. Touch your genitals and draw up
a sexual charge that's just for you.
- Fill yourself with glowing sensuality, ready to share.

A CALMING TEA

This tea will help you unwind from a busy day and clear the mind.

- First collect the herbs needed for your herbal tea: Lavender Flowers, Chamomile Flowers, Hops, Orange Peel, and Peppermint.
- Put 1 Tablespoon each of Hops and Chamomile into a sauce pan with 3 cups of boiling water.
- Add 1 teaspoon each of Lavender, chopped Orange Peel and Peppermint to the brew.
- Simmer for a few minutes.

It is done when the water has a slight change in color and the herbs in the water are quite soft and limp. It will be very aromatic. Add something for taste if desired... honey, maple syrup, lemon... it is up to you and your taste buds.

A MOVING MEDITATION
This beautiful meditation cleanses fatigue from body, mind and soul.

- Sit comfortably.
- Slow the pace of your breathing.
- Drop away from thought.
- Drop inside the breath, sending all of your awareness to its ebb and flow.
- Tune your awareness to the sensations the breath offers as it strokes your inner being.
- As held tension leaves the body/mind, open wholeheartedly to the joy of the present moment.
- Smile.
- Wiggle your sit bones deep into the earth, grounding, establishing a perfect fit.

𝐴. Place your hands at the base of your belly.

-Send your breath deep down to your hands, filling your body with subtle lift. As you exhale, follow the feeling of release and depth.

-Allow the breath to take your body with it in gentle sway, moving forward and with the pulse of each breath.

-Be here until you feel completely connected to the flow of your breath, the weight of your body, and the earth supporting below you.

Expand your awareness into the sensations available in this tiny but precious moment.

Stay here until all comes together as the feeling of peace.

B. Place your hands over your heart.

-Let your own warmth touch your heart with pure acceptance, compassion and loving care, rocking inside the arms of your breath.

-Be here until you feel soft, received, and at peace with yourself.

C. Rub your hands vigorously together.

-Feel a small flame growing between them.

-Place both hands gently over your face.

-Let your head rest forward into the warmth of your touch. Take nurture from your hands and peace from the darkness that draws your senses within to the eye of your calm.

-Release the weight of your head completely.

-Be here until you feel completely inside the sky of your mind.

D. Follow the next inhaled breath.

-Sweep your hands upward, stroking your forehead, brushing over your crown, and sweeping down the back of your head.

-Exhale. Interlace your fingers at the base of your skull and drop your elbows forward, gently drawing your chin toward your chest.

-Be here for several long slow cycles of breath, as tension leaves the neck and the long length of your spine.

E. Inhale, sitting up straight. Stretch your torso upward with the breath, lifting your heart and lifting your gaze.

-Exhale. Hang forward as before, talking several breaths in and out.

F. Release your fingers.

-Brush them down the sides of your head, traveling the length of your jaw in a slow stroke, off the chin and to your left, placing your right hand on your left knee and the fingertips of your left hand on the floor.

-Inhale. Slowly roll your head to your right shoulder.

-Exhale. Release the weight of your heavy head right, as you take support from your hands on the left. This opens up a nice river of release from your fingertips through your jaw.

-Stay here until all static impulse has given way to free flow.

Roll your chin to your chest and over to your left shoulder, as your hands move to your right, repeating this pause to the other side.

G. Roll your chin back to center.

-Lift your head and rock forward to stretch out in extended Child's Pose.

-Reach your hands as far forward as you can, while sending your hips back toward your heels.

-Drop the weight of your hips completely to the earth.

-Send your awareness to brush the long length of your back body, from fingertips to heels.

-Be heavier with each exhaled breath.

-Embrace gravity and descend.

-Hold here for several cycles of breath. Plant the seed of your gaze deep within, sending your inner eye to look back toward your navel.

H. Bend both arms at the elbows.

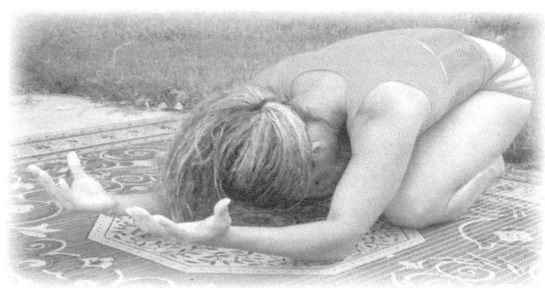

-Reach back to massage your neck and shoulders, squeezing tension out with your firm grip.

-Inhale big.

-Exhale strong, flying your hands forward to slap the ground, palms down, grounding the released energy and restoring balance.

-Repeat once more, massaging your neck and shoulders and "flicking the tension" away from your body.

I. Roll up like a big wave to sit back on your heels.

-Draw your hands up the midline of your body in one long stroke from your knees, over your abdomen, breast, throat and face.

-Continue upward, entwining your fingers with your hair to give it a firm but pleasant pull, increasing circulation through the scalp and freeing tension.

-Extend yourself into the continued feeling of upward moving life force.

-When ready, brush you hands down the back of your head,

forward along your jaw, across your chest, sliding down the ribs and off of your buttocks, planting your palms firmly to either side of your feet.

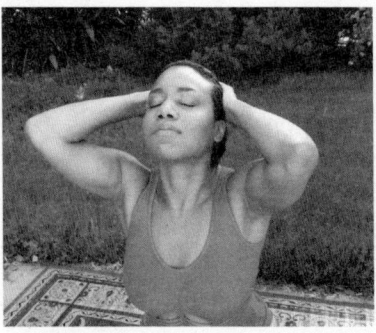 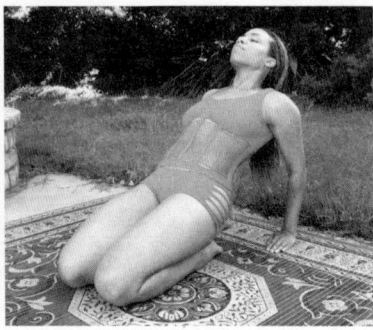

J. Inhale, lifting your thighs, hips and heart toward the sky, your front body open to life.

-Exhale, lowering your hips to your heels and bowing low in Child's Pose.

-You can increase the release through your shoulders by clasping your hands behind your back and bringing them up and overhead as your upper body spills forward over your lap.

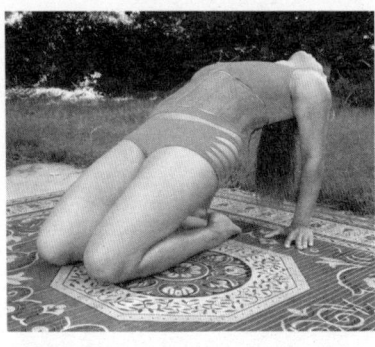 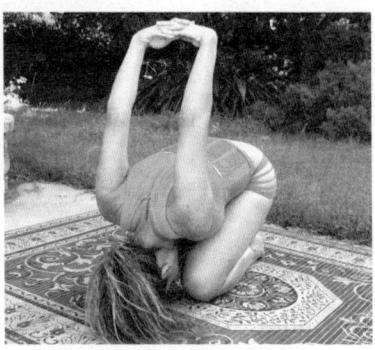

Return to seated, rolling up like a big wave to sit on your heels.

Repeat *J.*

𝒦. Use your hands for support and hop your feet beneath your hips.

-With fingertips on the floor, straighten your legs and move to a relaxed Forward Bend.

𝓛. Standing Breath of Joy

-Hang forward, inviting deep rest.
-Pour the entire weight of your upper body out of your hips, a waterfall free and flowing, filling your reservoirs with fresh life force.

-Place your hands back to back and slowly rise one vertebra at a time. Your fingertips follow, drawing a plumb line directly through center, tracing inner calves and thighs, brushing your sex and abdomen, cresting your heart and
lifting your chin.

-Reach to touch the sky in one long yawning flow of breath and awareness that spans from your fingertips to your toes. Continue to...

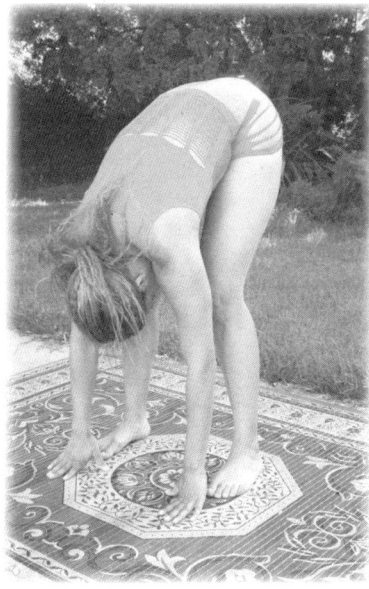
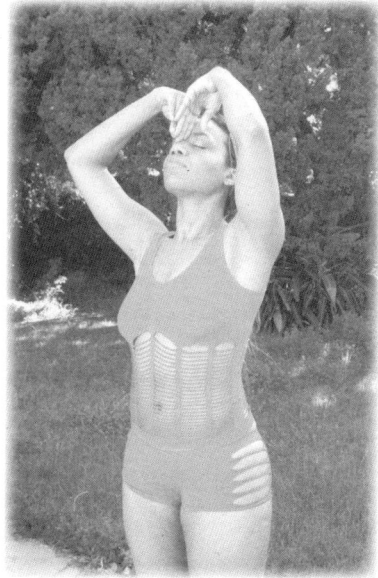

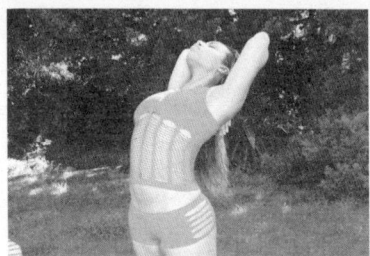

Lean slightly back as your hands rotate, turning palm to palm. Bend your arms at the elbows to touch the back of your heart with awakening. ➡

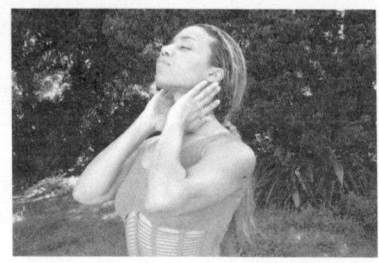

Flow your hands forward as before, past ears and jaw, over the heart and down your sides...

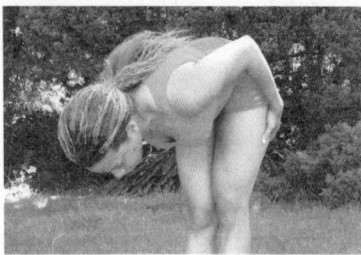

sweeping around your hips to travel from top of your buttocks...

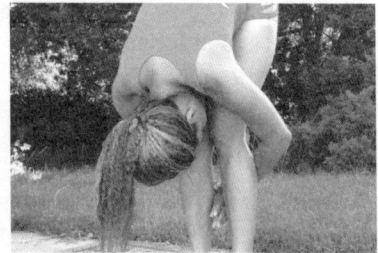

to the foundation of your feet, as a divine blessing proffered from the heart of your hands.

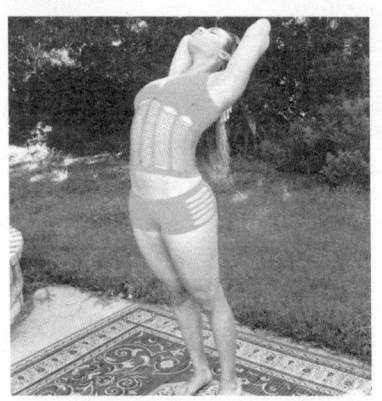

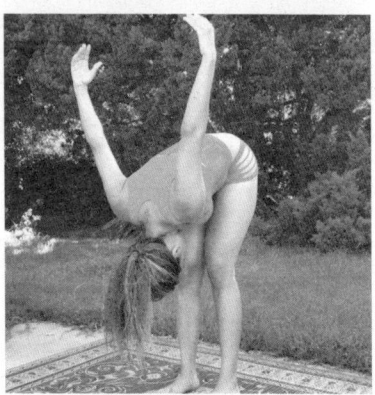

Inhale. Body and fingers follow the same trail in rising up to touch the sky. Exhale as a powerful release, playfully swinging your hands, head and upper body forward and down in one great whoosh. Inhale. Swing up and exhale release. Repeat entire Standing Breath of Joy cycle.

M. Rolling around: a series of little hugs.

-From Forward Bend, lower yourself to sit cross legged on the floor.

-Rest your cheek against your right knee and nestle into your own warmth. Be like a little bird sleeping beneath its wing, safe and secure.

-Rest for several breaths.

-Roll to your left and onto your back.

-Pull your knees in to your chest, hugging them close.

-Rock side to side. Be a cradle, rocking and soothing yourself.

-Roll to your right, coming back to seated. Nestle once again with your left cheek to your left knee.

-Move to completion, coming to center and folding forward in utter surrender. Rest your forehead to floor or take ease with a pillow.

-With your hands palm to palm, extend your Namaste to the divinity within.

Upon rising, sit quietly for a few moments.

Absorb the effect of the gift you have given to yourself. Observe the change in your thoughts, emotions, energy, and body.

Gaze into your peace as it unfolds from within.

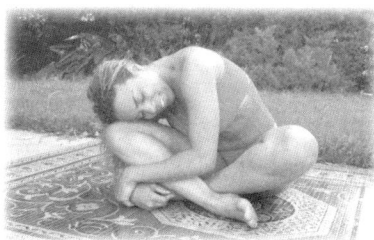
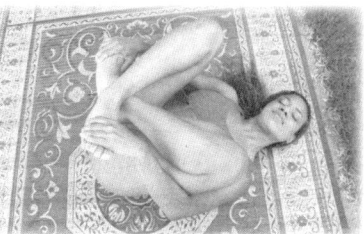

Chapter 2: Sanctuary - Setting the Scene
Making a Place for Practice

Choosing a place to practice erotic yoga is a treat to be shared. The conscious act of making a space that feels sexy, warm and inviting is a first step toward bringing yourselves into alignment with each other.

Your place of practice may be simple. An empty space can be easily transformed into a sanctuary set apart with a soft rug, overstuffed pillows, and gentle candlelight. Simplicity itself can evoke a feeling of tranquility and ease. For those who love ceremony, the possibilities are endless in creating a room made specifically for pleasure.

Choose elements that appeal to your senses and inspire your spirit. Make a weaving of colors, smells, sights and sounds that arouse your sensuality and invite peace. As you search for the elements that will make your purr-fect environment, you will find multiple resources in the beauty of our world culture and the abundance of the earth.

Go on a sensual scavenger hunt with your partner. Take a walk and keep your eyes open for anything that speaks to your senses. A ticklish feather or a smooth river stone can be used to soothe or excite, becoming Shaman's tools in your loving hands. Strands of ivy, rose petals or any available flower will add a special touch of imagination to your time together. You may never be able to look at a pussy willow again with a straight face.

A thunder drum, Tibetan singing bowl or temple gong can mark the entry to your world between the worlds, clearing the air with pure vibration.

Make magic with candles anointed with oils, scent and color... released with lusty intention. Fill the room with an ocean of sultry sounds, finding music that moves you both. Poetry books for inspired words can add an aura of devotional light.

Anchor your foundation to the four directions by filling your corners with the elements of sympathetic magic, which means choosing something similar to the mood, atmosphere and feeling you wish to create.

Just as the yoga postures and chakras are tied to the five elements, each direction has its own significance, for example:

Light incense to your East. Air - the element representing knowledge/Illumination.

Light fire to your South. Fire - the element representing vitality/power.

To your West, pour water in a reflective bowl. Water - the element representing subconscious emotions and the fluidity of change.

To the North, lay a beautiful stone as Earth - the element representing all of nature and your place within it, her presence enduring as a witness to all life. Here in your space, ask for the gift of silence, and the craft of deep listening.

Lay out your room as a sacred symbol.

Make a moving meditation of your actions and thoughts when in that space. Feel every object as potent with positive emotional charge, and every footstep as one taken the direction of intimate trust. Your space holds the imprint of your loving connection, giving it a quality of presence unlike any other.

As you build your Sanctuary together, you are laying a foundation of personal meaning crystal by crystal, and stone by stone, rediscovering what is hot and what is not. Find what moves you and go with it.

Let ceremony and ritual flow from the heart of your own mystery to speak to one another. Set the scene and play it out.

You have made a nest, a hiding place, a gateway from the ordinary to the sublime. Who could say "no" to an invitation like this?

Chapter 3: Opening Salutation/Meditation
Honoring one Another - Recognition

Your first touch actually happens before either of you lays a tender hand upon the other.

It is all about energy - a look, a smile, a soft word, a sigh. The words "Come here," uttered with just the right tone, can practically rip the clothes off of some of us, while a direct look from heavy-lidded "bedroom eyes" will undo the rest. These energetic cues create a powerful response in magnetizing one to another, based on past experience of the pleasure that followed acceptance of the command.

As you come together, it is nice to share an intimate greeting, finding a personal and meaningful way to receive your partner. Remember that secret handshake you had for your closest friend as a child? Those series of claps, high fives and fist bumps acknowledged a bond that no one else could entirely share. Put some playful thought into creating a first touch that calls out to the passionate lover in each of you. Your ritual greeting - be it a deep kiss and an ear nibble, or simply letting your eyes rest on your partner's face - sends the message *"Here I Am,"* through the soul of your gaze.

Once found, hold your words and actions as sacred, set apart, and consecrated for this use and this use alone. Your greeting will become imbued with power... a ritual taking on special significance and deeper meaning each time you meet, and becoming charged with the vibration of your whole practice as pleasures past enliven your present response.

A gesture or word in itself is empty, but with the life force of trained awareness behind them, your practiced touch will hold enough energy to trigger a shift in consciousness.

Use your greeting to move your relaxed sense of *I Am* outward, to flow through the expanding framework of *We Are*. We bring "I am here" into "Here I am," bathed in the light of pure acceptance. Heart-centered love frees each other to receive without fear, and to give without withholding, all streams flowing into the same ocean and the experience you share.

Aladdin said "Open Sesame," and the great rocks slid apart. Your "Here I Am," intoned with both a depth of soul and your firm hands to his hard body, can move the sentry stones from the cave of the heart. It can reveal treasure rare, along with the God/Goddess within, whose gift it is to give.

In finding your ritual greeting, the best way will ultimately emerge from the heart of your relationship and add a dimension of romance and fun. Remember, laughter is another great stress buster and a real smile is a real turn-on.

A few greetings to get you started in cultivating a new awareness of one another:

1. Namaste

"Namaste" is a beautiful Hindu word which carries the powerful vibration of divine recognition.

To extend Namaste through spoken word and gentle bow, with your hands pressed palm to palm before the heart, indicates a stance or posture of the spirit. It says "I bow to you," or "I bow to the divine within you," speaking to the truth of our unity in the light of divine consciousness. We are all one.

This creates a simple greeting ritual by adapting the concept of the mudra - which refers to symbolic gestures usually held with the fingers - to include the whole body in crafting a gesture of love, honor and divine recognition.

Begin by coming close together, offering the shelter of your body as a safe resting place.

- Find a comfortable whole body hug that gives maximum support and snug body contact, creating a "mudra" of your entwined bodies. Include a special way to seal your hands to further express your unspoken wish.

- Hold each other closer, your breathing rhythmic, your hearts slow, and your edges soft.

- Melt and merge your hearts together with each breath, expanding and opening to make a mudra of
your hearts as one heart.

- Be alive to the divinity you hold in your arms.

- Be awake to the divinity that lives within your heart.

- Stretch out. Reach into the joy of your soul.

- Dissolve in the sweetness of your deepest hug. Sizzle with the gift of passion in your embrace.

~Namaste~

Use Namaste alone or weave its enormous spirit and abundant warmth into your practice with the following phrase:

> With all the strength of my body
> With all the love of my heart
> With all the light of my mind
> I celebrate the divinity within you
> With all the joy of my soul
> ~Namaste~

Invent your own body language, touch, and gestures to further express the feeling.

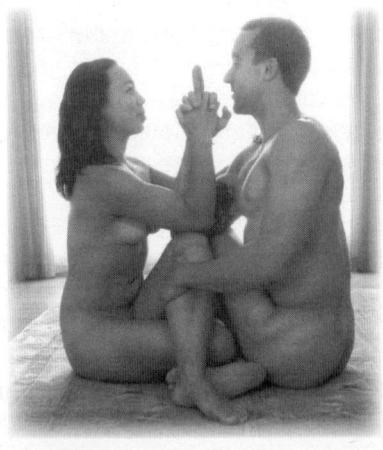

Chapter 4: Pranayamas
A Sensual Point of View

Just as a desert blooms with the gift of falling rain, we seize life with the gift of our first breath, a divine kiss drawing forth the flower of our spirit.

Pranayamas are specific breathing exercises that are central to the practice of yoga. The purpose of the practice is revealed by its name: "prana" meaning life force, and "yama" meaning control. The careful practice of breath control, along with the Asanas (the physical postures of yoga), direct the flow of your life force energy much the way a river's banks channel its power in one focused direction. In a pranayama practice, your mind and the breathing techniques you will learn provide banks of awareness that direct the raw energy of your life force to a refined and potent focus.

To connect with your breath is to fully enter into a conscious partnership with your life force.

Proper breath control Pranayama is an essential part of a yoga routine. It keeps the mind clear and the body steady during the physical practice of yoga postures and is a form of meditation with an extra punch. Each pranayama contains a highly specific series of breaths. The number of inhalations and exhalations, as well as the speed of each breath, opens the flow of energy and awareness to invite the desired effect.

Coupled with awakening self awareness, the exercises are organized to affect your state of mind and restore health and vitality to the organs and glands of your body. The yogic breath, once learned, can add staying power to your lovemaking sessions and stir up longer stronger orgasms... the cherry on top of a luscious experience.

As we seek a sense of deeper union, a shared meditation on the breath draws the life force of one into harmony with that of the other. Breathing in unison opens complimentary currents of energy that connect the fine network of our extended energy fields like curious fingers finding one another between the sheets. As you become comfortable with the basic yogic breath you will begin to experience it as another dimension of self that is as much a part of you as your emotions and thoughts - another dimension of touch that runs through and beyond the physical body as an intimate sensual stroke.

In essence, the breath shared in unison with your partner becomes another form of making love. There is a deep sense of a penetration and the beautiful sigh of letting go, both leaving a tingly thrill and the promise of more.

Dropping into the river of each breath and following its sensual flow, we begin to generate an endlessly intimate caress that is felt on multiple levels: thoughts, emotions, heartbeat and pulse, body heat and growing arousal. All move into sizzling alignment. Don't underestimate the power of something as commonplace as your breath to become a favorite aphrodisiac. With yogic awareness and a little well-placed control, this weaving of life force one to another is intimate and enlightening, offering a more complete sense of merger than a physical penetration alone.

Begin with a few simple exercises that highlight a sense of full connectivity or true union, to do both solo and with your partner. Prana (life force) yama (control) is another step on the path we will follow into the expanse of each others' open hearts.

The Pranayamas

I approach pranayamas with a sense of awe and devotion. They are magical... bridging body, mind and spirit with a simple grace that allows all to enter.

The traditional pranayamas are very powerful and to be used with care and the instruction of a patient teacher.

We are exploring variations of the basic yoga breath to support your most intimate connection through meditation, touch, and movement.

For our purposes, the breath now becomes a medium for deepening contact and extending our awareness as a form of touch.

Together, these exercises form one full practice that constitutes a "work out" for your prana/energy and awareness, leaving your mind clear and your body receptive.

We offer five simple breath experiences as the foundation for all that follows.

1. Basic Yogic Breath - Seated
All begins with a quiet mind, gently following the journey of the breath.
- Sit comfortably face to face or back to back.
- Inhale naturally.
- Exhale, relaxing.

Breathing through your nostrils, continue in soft natural rhythm while tuning your awareness to the full length and feeling of each breath.

- Notice where the breath starts and where it ends.
- Notice its character and quality. Is it shallow or deep? Steady or uneven?
- Listen with your whole body. Be curious - become absorbed.
- Under your gentle gaze, each breath will gradually stretch out - becoming long, lazy and relaxed.
- Inhale as if filling the ocean from its floor, following its swell to touch the sky.
- Exhale as a cloud releases rain: Pour.

Continue in this pattern until you feel peace enfolding you in its arms.

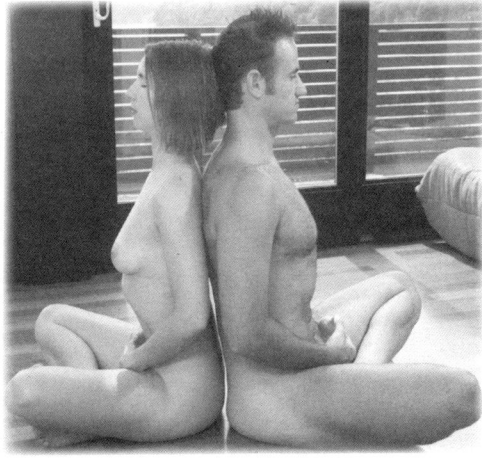

All of the following exercises can be done using the basic breath as their foundation.

If you want another level of inward focus and tranquility, you may add:

2. Ujjayi Breathing or Ocean-Sounding Breath

The distinct sound of Ujjayi breath is likened to the sound of the sea in ebb and flow. Another name for this breathing pattern is "Ocean-Sounding Breath."

- Breathe in and out through the nose.

- Lightly constrict the back of the throat making it feel a little tight, the same way it does when you try to whisper "Hey" loudly enough to be heard by someone across a room.

Maintain that same feeling while keeping your lips closed and continuing to breathe in and out through the nostrils.

This subtle action in the throat creates the distinctive Ujjayi sound as the narrowed airway creates slight resistance, slowing each breath down.

The slower breath causes more oxygen to be absorbed into the blood and by the brain.

Practice this breath seated comfortably until it becomes natural... easy... without effort.

When you are adept at using the Ujjayi breath seated, you can use it to keep the body steady and the mind clear while practicing yoga postures... or... while making love, enhancing a sense of shared connection.

Using Basic Yogic Breath or Ujjayi Breathing, continue on.

3. Shared Breath

Now extend your awareness to reach your partner, expanding from your own sense of center to move just beyond the boundaries of your skin.

- Sit back to back.
- Root your sit bones into the cushion of the Earth below.
- Press your backs together, both offering and being support to one another.

Attune to the presence of each breath, its flight when taken, and its fall in release. Feel your backs expand into one another as you inhale, and relax into one another as you exhale, becoming close with each cycle of breath.

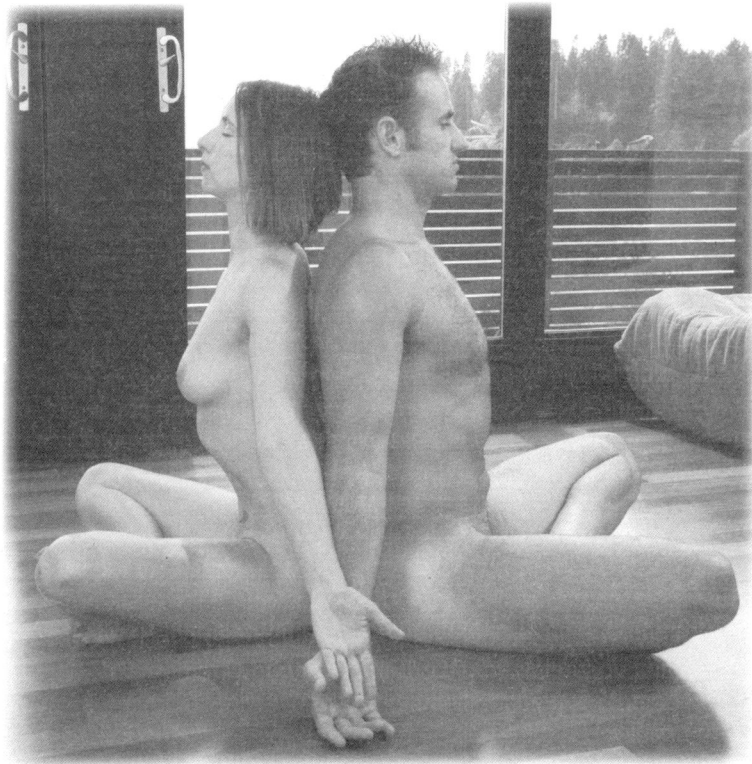

- Listen to the sound of your breaths in harmony... a sound like a flowing river.

- Sit by the river side, observing. Cast your mind into the flow.

- Let yourselves fall in and be swept away.

- Become the current, the sound, the energy.

- Become the part of you that IS the breath.

As your breathing falls together, two become one.

This simple merger of focus, action and energy establishes a tangible current of pure connection.

4. Sending Breath – Give and Receive
Turn face to face. Move in close. Wrap your legs around each other's hips and snuggle into a loose hug.

- Inhale. Imagine drawing the breath in through your crown and filling yourself completely.

- Exhale all the way down through your sit bones, rooting yourself to the earth below.

Let the energy of the breath carry you. Become absorbed in its rise and fall. Once the breath and the visualization are established, move your awareness to your genitals - the area of the second chakra.

- Inhale as if through the crown.

- Exhale, expanding warm awareness though your sexual center outward toward you partner.

As you send - so you receive. This is a simultaneous touch - an infinity loop of giving which becomes receiving all in one breath.

As you exhale, imagine a part of you reaching forward - touching, tasting, caressing, inhabiting your partner. Feel the loving tendrils of awareness flowing from your partner into you. Let yourself drop beyond thought and into the feelings without picking them apart. In other words BE in the moment. Just this one, here and now. Stay inside this focus for a few minutes.

Notice how your genitals feel. Are they warm? Juicy? Tingly? Alive?

Do these feelings move to any other area of your body?

Do you feel fully connected to your genitals and your sensuality?

- Breathe deeper.

- Move your awareness upward to the Heart chakra and continue to open to your partner and yourself for a few more minutes.

- When you are both ready, return the focus to your crown, or Sahasrara, chakra and take in a clearing breath.

- Exhale down through your roots, grounding the experience in the earthy foundation of the whole body.

This creates a strong sense of give and take while bringing a unity of mind, breath and body. In this pattern we can feel the invisible circuitry of our wireless anatomy begin to hum.

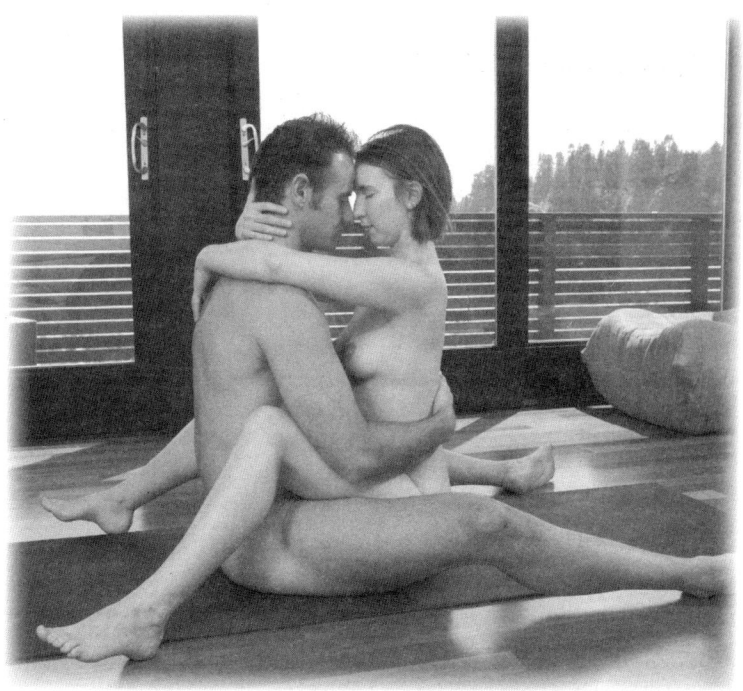

Moola Bhanda

- Exhale slowly. Imagine riding an elevator down to the basement floor.

- Relax into the firm connection of your lower body with the earth. Feel your sit bones rooted to the floor. Relax your hips and buttocks.

- Draw your awareness to the area between your anus and your genitals/perineum. Note any sensations there.

We will call this the ground floor of the body. In practicing Moola Bandha, this area becomes the place to draw awareness and energy upward from, and our steady point of return.

- As you inhale, imagine moving back up to the first, second and third floor, while drawing the muscles around the perineum up and in.

- Hold here, retaining the breath for 6 to 10 counts before slowly returning to the ground floor with your relaxed exhalation.

- Use steady control throughout. The sensation here can be likened to holding back the flow of urine, or trying to stop it midstream, before relaxing again.

- As you continue to practice, notice the area between your genitals, anus, and perineum becoming alive with sensation. Follow the sensual feelings that Moola Bandha brings as it puts you directly in touch with the sexual core of your body.

-Add little Pelvic Tilts to deepen the flow of the breath and pleasurable sensations as you begin to awaken your erotic energies from within: softly roll your pelvis forward as you inhale and back as you exhale in tiny Cat Stretch-like movements.

Practice this exercise often and you will be rewarded. It will strengthen and tone the vaginal walls after childbirth and aid in reversing incontinence. The practice encourages blood flow through the vagina - making you more sensitive during sex - as well as introducing you to your ability to tighten and relax the vaginal walls when making love.

This tightening and letting go will increase your pleasure, and your partner's, as you can draw his penis deeply inside with gentle massage-like squeezes. You can also make firmer contact with his penis as he penetrates - doubling your pleasure all the way around... a win/win situation.

Practice Moola Bandha before making love. Start with 1 minute and slowly increase to 10 minutes. Draw your awareness to what you feel, sense, and receive from this personally intimate practice. Revel in your own sexual energy rising. Once you have Moola Bhanda under your belt, keep on exploring!

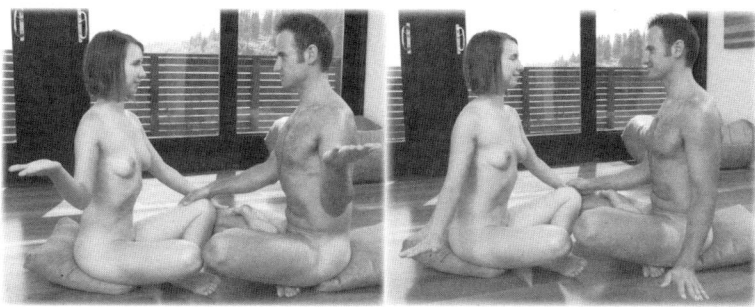

5. Inverted Breath

Use breath 3, filling completely and sending through your sexual center but passing the breath back and forth in circular cycles.
- She inhales while he exhales.
- He inhales while she exhales.
- One breath pours into the other.

Feel the strong sense of connection, your life forces weaving together in one strong current, two halves of one inseparable whole.

Making it deeper:

- Continue to invite a supercharged sense of closeness.

- From seated face to face, extend your legs forward toward one another.

- Bend your knees and place your feet a hip width apart while lying down on your backs. You will each plant your feet to the outside of your partner's hips and then relax your knees outward.

- Continue with the Inverted Breath.

- He inhales, rolling his pelvis forward, low back lifting from the floor, while...

- She exhales, drawing her tailbone up and under, pressing her low back to the floor.

- Now HE exhales, drawing his tailbone up and under, while...

- She inhales, rolling her pelvis forward, low back lifting from the floor.

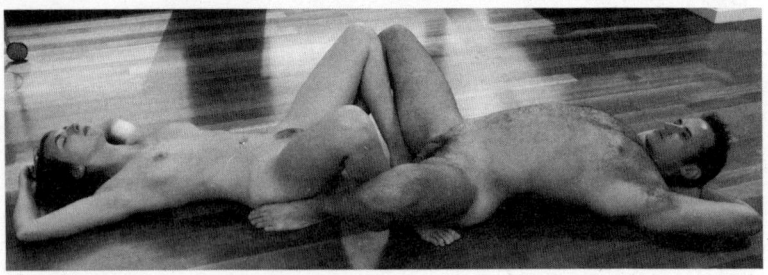

The practice creates a slow steady wave of unbroken connection, much like making love. The posture and the focus of your awareness will revitalize your sex organs, bringing fresh circulation through the pelvis and groin as well as melting tensions held in the hips and low back.

Now that you are in touch with the sensual nature of the breath and the complete sense of connection it brings, add a partnered flow of gentle strokes and stretches.

Moving Meditations for Two

PRACTICE 1 – A PLAYFUL WARM UP

EXERCISE KEY ◉ ○ ●
◉ Moving in unison
○ Partner 1
● Partner 2

Basic Yogic Breath Revisited
This combination of Deep Breath and motion invites you to unwind together while freeing your hips, back and spine from tension.

◉ Sit cross legged, face to face.
◉ Fall into the Deep Breath.
◉ Fall into harmony with your partner.
◉ Wait for a sense of connection to arrive.
◉ Allow the breath to become effortless, guided by the body instead of the mind.

◉ Inhale, elongating your spine and stretching your torso up out of your hips.
◉ Exhale, folding forward one at a time to Closed Lotus Pose.
○ Fold forward, wrapping your arms around his waist or legs, cheek nesting on the pillow of his inner thigh.
● Fold over her body, stroking her back as you find your way down, taking her into the shelter of your arms.
◉ Stay here for 3 full cycles of breath - a closed lotus bud awaiting the time to bloom.

◉ Release the pose slowly, rising to place your hands to each other's shoulders.
◉ Begin to circle to your right, sustaining a deep even breath throughout the cycle.
◉ Circle right 5 times and pause, returning to Closed Lotus Pose.
● Fold forward to rest your cheek against her thigh.
○ Follow with a warm caress to rest over his body.

◉ Pause for 3 full cycles of breath before rising.

◉ Now circle left for five long breaths.

◉ Repeat once more to each side.

◉ To finish, bring your circling to center and rest your hands over your partner's heart.

Continue to breath in deep even flow.

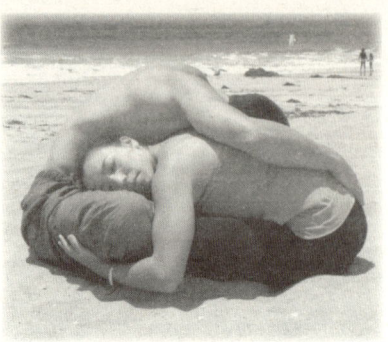

SEATED CAT STRETCH

◉ With your palms warmly on your partner's, inhale, flexing your spine and sending your heart toward your partner. It is nice to move cheek to cheek.

◉ Exhale. Powerfully round your back while releasing the breath, your hands stroking down the length of the arms to hold firmly above the wrists.

◉ Continue to take the breath in and out, each breath supporting the length of each movement - your whole spine dancing in flex and arch, your whole body absorbing prana.

◉ Follow the ascendant arc of light with your inner eye and spirit body. Repeat 7 times.

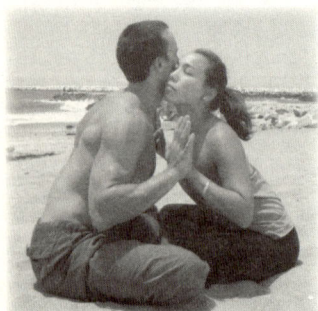
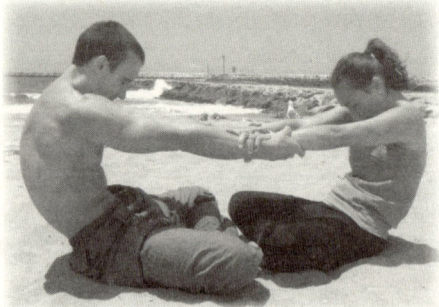

INNER TEMPLE

◉ Return to center and lean forward, arms overhead, hands palm to palm. Rest your heads together, eye to eye, following your gaze inside the soul.

◉ Release the pose slowly, your hands full of healing light. Slide from crown down the back in a flowing stroke, sealing yourselves inside the circle of your arms.

◉ Return to center.

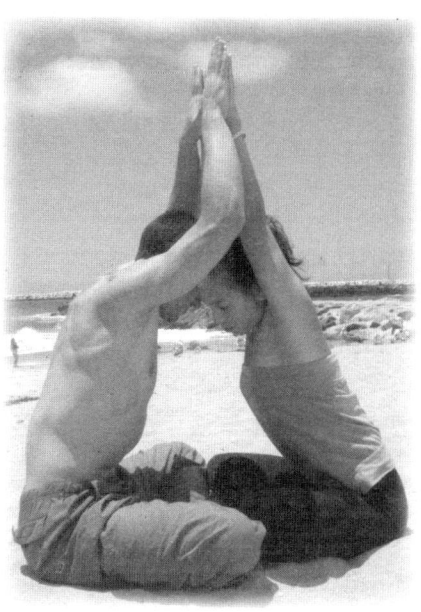

SIMPLE TWIST

◉ Fold your right arm behind your lower back.

Reach out with your left hand to find your partner's right hand.

Inhale, elongating your spine as you fill from bottom to top.

Exhale to your right into the twist. Send your chin in the same direction.

Hold here for several cycles of breath before repeating to your left.

ENTWINED HUG

◉ Come to center and extend both legs forward to either side of your partner's hips. Scooch close enough to bend your knees and rest your feet together behind your partner's back.

◉ Get close, and closer still, pressing the front of your bodies together in unbroken contact.

◉ Settle into the warmth of this hug, wrapping your arms completely around each other's backs.

◉ Fall into...

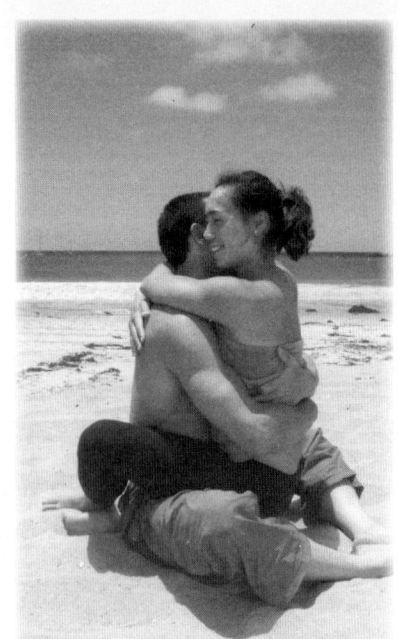

THE SENDING BREATH

◉ Inhale, filling through the crown of your head to light up every cell of your body.

◉ Exhale through your sexual center, sending your self through your partner.

In this "exercise" we let the breath speak for itself.

- Feel the deepening sense of merger as giving and receiving become one action.

- Gradually follow the thread of the inhaled breath to pierce the center of each glowing chakra.

- Exhale, sending forth rays from the heart of each charka to meet your partner in effusive warmth.

Breathe, Melt, Be……

- Feel the growing light and heat inside you.

- Imagine your hearts burning as one candle flame. Follow the glow. Let go of the mind and try it.

Be here for as long as you wish. Now move again to...

INVERTED BREATH
- Inhale long and slow.
- Exhale deeply and evenly.
- Continue on until the pattern is natural and without much thought or effort.

If you are ready for more in-depth practice, add Moola Bhanda every few cycles of breath to continue to juice up your sex organs. Feel the sacred fire of your delicious sexuality rising.

- Focus on the circular nature of the energies flowing through you.
- Follow the sensation with the interest of your body and enter the circle with your will, wish, and imagination - part of you flowing inside the golden loop of prana weaving its way through your total being.
- Take firm hold of your partner's hips.
- Flex your spine when you inhale and round your back when you exhale. This gently raises latent forces sleeping in the cradle of the sacrum, a pleasing rocking motion that is reminiscent of making love.

- Continue on in pleasurable exchange, the inverted breath becoming effortless, taking time to fall into your natural rhythm.

- As you inhale, imagine drawing in your partner's exhaled breath to circulate as light all the way through your inner circuitry to meet the life force resident inside of your sex.

- As you exhale, imagine giving your energy inside the flow of breath to your partner. Give from the heart of your heat - from one to another. Drink in the energy offered through the genitals. Pull it upward to the third eye and back down again. Move it through your sex to your partner in an unbroken cycle, pouring into each other from an infinite source.

OPENING TO LOVE

◙ When you feel ready, slip your hands around your partner's lower back.

○ Let go and let him support you totally. As you lean back, your heart is freed to expand to a place of freedom and trust.

• Follow her forward with your whole upper body. As her back meets the ground, release both of your hands to brush up the mid line of her body with your hands in a warm sweeping gesture.

• Sit up slowly, leaving her at rest as your hands brush down the length of her arms to her fingertips.

• Repeat 3 times, pulling her up to seated on the last repetition.

◙ Return to the Inverted Breath with your hands around your partner's low back. Wait for 3 cycles of breath before repeating all for the other partner.

◙ Follow the exchange to its end.

◙ Rest seated in warm embrace.

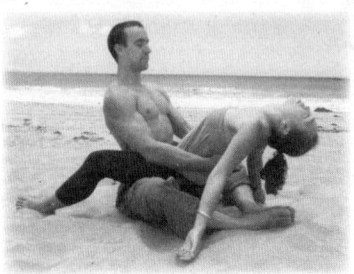
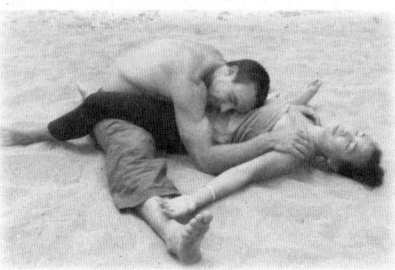

PRACTICE 2 – A NURTURING EXCHANGE

CIRCLING THE SEA
○ Sit comfortably, cross legged on the floor.

• Kneel behind her. Separate your knees and draw her close.

• Wrap your arms around her belly.

○ Wrap your arms over his.

◙ On the rhythm of the breath, inhale, leaning slightly back and to the right. Then exhale, circling forward and to your left, making a large circle of one cycle of breath.

Repeat 3 times.

Repeat 3 times in the opposite direction, circling left.

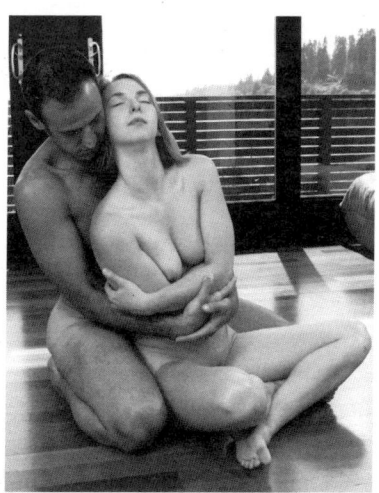

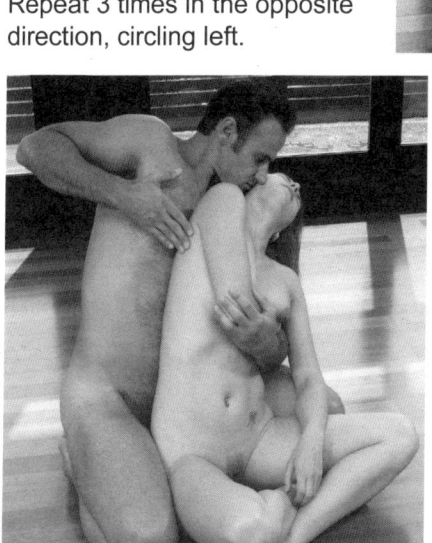

SOOTHING SIGH
◙ Inhale fully.

◙ Exhale, leaning to your left side.
• Stroke your hand down her right side from her highest ribs to her buttocks.
• Inhale, returning to center as your fingertips lightly brush back up her side.
◙ Repeat 3 times before shifting to the other side.

FLYING HOME
◙ Wrap your arms around the heart center.
◙ Inhale, flexing your spine, lifting your eyes and drawing the arms wide open, as if flying into the face of the sun.
◙ Exhale, dropping your chin to your chest, rounding your back and folding your arms over your chest, sheltering in the shadow of your wings.

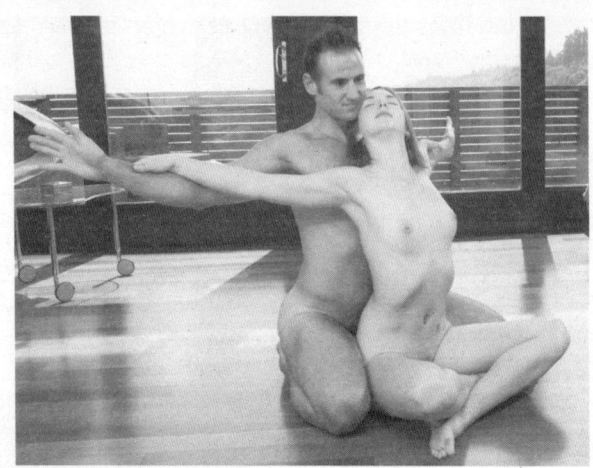

A TWISTED KISS
- Kneel behind her, making your posture snug.

- Lift your right hand up and over in a big arch-like movement, twisting to kiss your partner.

- Repeat in the opposite direction, lifting your left hand.

- Follow gravity forward and down, like water pouring over a stone. Let yourselves pour out, running free.

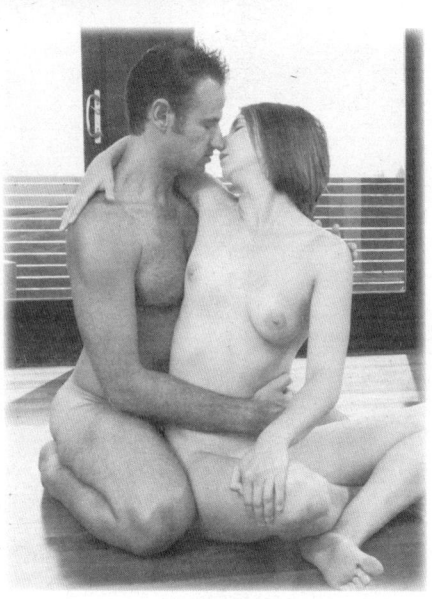

PLANK POSE
- Softly fold your body over hers, or lean in deep. Plant your palms on the floor, your chest, abdomen and thighs resting on her back. Your toes tucked under carry the rest of your weight.

- Massage her back and shoulders as you release the pose.

Rest together.

Turn, exchanging roles from active to passive and repeat for the other partner.

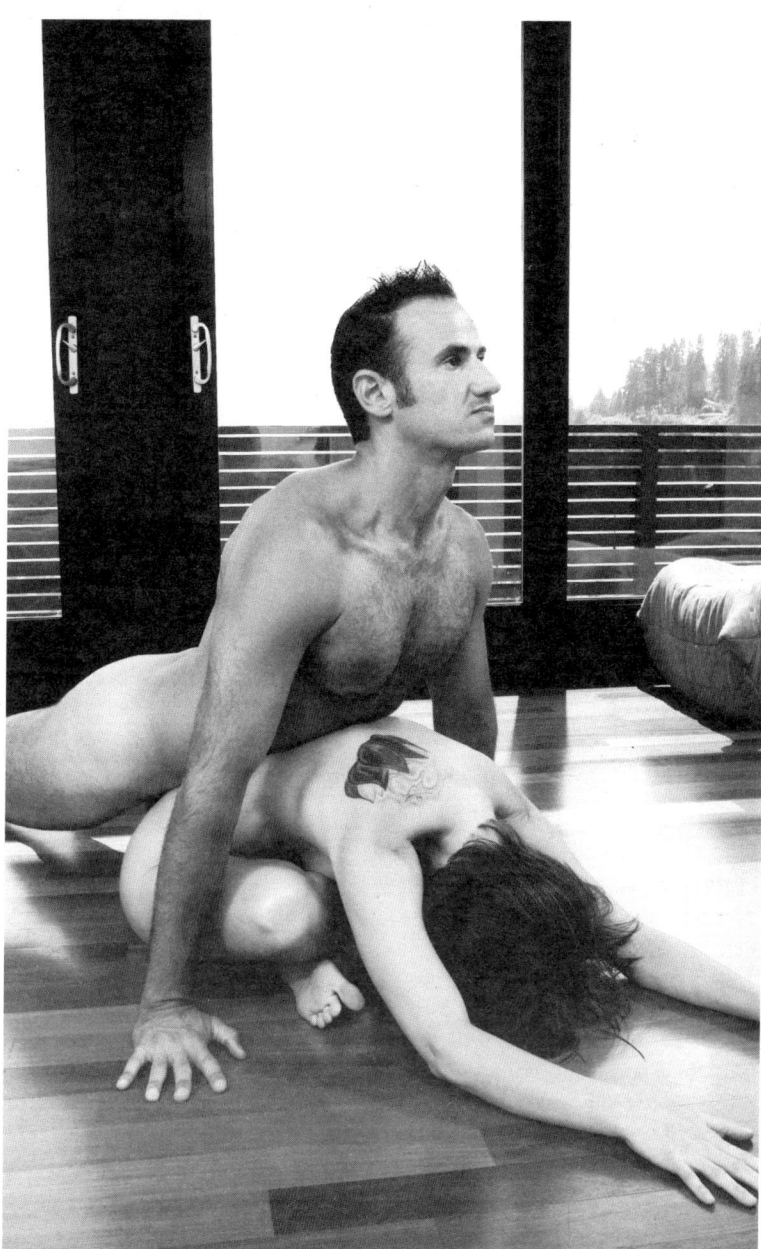

Chapter 5: Basic Meditation
Clearing the Head and Heart

"Keep your head in the game" is another way of saying "Be Here Now."

After all, when you are making love the last thing you need to be doing is making a mental shopping list for dinner or worrying over the late fee on your last DVD rental. It is hard to be a great lover if your thoughts are somewhere else. To this end we recommend an opening and a closing meditation.

Why meditate?

Meditation is a detoxification program for the mind which will leave you with a clear head and an open heart. Simply put, a meditation practice clears the mind of clutter.

The object of meditation is not so much to empty the mind or to silence all thoughts, but to create clarity by training the mind to one pure focus. A single focus on a single activity will invite a calm place of peaceful awareness. Most meditation practices center on following the breath as it comes and goes.

Inhale - Here.
Exhale - Now.

Work with the principle of "Nothing Extra." Follow one breath at a time - just the breath - one breath lowing into the next in seamless cycles. When you follow the sensation of the breath you will find an abundance of enticing feelings to observe:

The breath is cool when it comes in through your nostrils and warm when it leaves.

Your inhalation has a light upward sensation. The exhalation feels grounding and deep.

All of these sensations gently seal your mind to a singular focus - the breath. Just each breath with nothing else attached. No action or reaction. Nothing Extra.

Leave your mental baggage behind and enlighten up.

Sitting in meditation is like hitting the Reset button on your computer. The brain has a chance to clear.

Meditation allows the mind to rest and renew itself. Instead of being caught up in the endless barrage of external stimulate, we engage the mind with its own resonant hum. We tap into our own consciousness as pure energy, limitless space, and endless potential. It is here that the mind expands to a regenerative non-reactive state. It is in this state that we can find deep peace and expansive joy. The reset button isn't where you thought. It is where you think.

As easy as it might sound, sitting in meditation takes some practice. The mind is easily distracted and is masterful at creating distraction. For most of us, the first thing that happens when we try to meditate is that we become aware of how insanely busy our thought life is. Random images, conversations, things you'd rather be doing or the dull ache in your lower back will beg for your attention. You may find your mind is a wild horse, balking at any hint of being saddled up and told where to go. Our thoughts, like wild horses, need to be trained, reined in and compassionately redirected to one chosen destination. Your meditation practice will give you the reins and become the destination.

As beginners, let's not expect an empty mind. Instead we will get acquainted with our favorite distractions.

Your first lesson in meditation is this: Sit and observe your thoughts. That's right, observe them. You cannot force a mind to be still. Just try it. Go ahead, be tough. Tell yourself that you are going to sit down and be quiet. Try to impose silence and see what happens. Most likely a lot of inner chatter will defiantly rise to the challenge. So watch and learn. Meet each thought for a moment. Do not follow it to the next idea but take a deep breath and let go. Sit with just your breathing as company until the next thought arrives. Treat each thought as a temporary guest to acknowledge and release.

Having become masterful at observing your thoughts you are now in a position to redirect them by actively listening to the breath. A simple focus on the breath is one way to call your wandering thoughts back to a place called NOW... Now being a place of wholeness that is without need or want.

When we think and act from a place of wholeness, all of our relationships benefit.

The Nature of the Breath
Breathing brings us into rhythm with all things.

Its steady cycles of Inhale/expand and Exhale/contract are reflected in the sound of waves to the shore, the ebb and flow of the tides, the cycles of the moon, and the routine miracle of another day following a good night's rest. Without the breath, we are disconnected from life; through the breath we participate with all life.

When the breath is unsteady all is unsteady. When the breath is smooth and even, your emotions, mind and actions will reflect the same tranquil quality. When we rest our gaze upon the breath, we become absorbed, purifying our thoughts with this singular focus.

The mind becomes open, spacious and clear as the breath itself creates balance and harmony between the systems of the body and the activity of the mind.

To begin:

- Sit upright in a comfortable position and breathe naturally.
- Close your eyes and allow your senses to follow the breath as it comes and goes.
- Breathe in and out through your nostrils.
- Focus on the subtle feeling of the breath as it meets your nostrils - it is cooling.
- Follow the breath as it flows out through your nostrils - it is warm.
- Continue to follow the breath by feeling not thinking.
- What is there to feel?... to absorb through all your senses?
- Gradually allow each breath to lengthen and deepen, becoming slow and relaxed.
- Imagine the breath to be the first or the last you may ever take.
- Relish every sweet moment.
- Be Here.
- Be Now.

- Dive in deep... stay inside the current.
- Let the breath take you, instead of you taking a breath.
- Smile.

As you practice, you will be learning to meditate while developing an ultra-charged sense of receptivity to subtle sensations. With practice, you will find that you can enjoy this same heightened awareness while riding the bigger waves of erotic/orgasmic energies to a longer stronger finish.

In your loving, the breath becomes an amazingly intimate exchange that is infused with extraordinary awareness. The feeling, the sound, the ebb and flow of your bodies in motion, your sighs and whispers all create union between spirit and matter, mind and body, inner space and outer limits.

For another level of focus add a mantra. Mantras are a highly specific series of syllables and sounds that draw the mind and spirit to a defined focus. Just the way you tune to a favorite radio station to put you in the right mood with the right playlist, a mantra dials the brain in to a specific vibration or channel. The feeling of tuning in is unmistakable, as all your inner static fades away.

One translation for the word mantra is "The thought that liberates or protects." A mantra liberates you from destructive thinking patterns and protects you from further negativity. Just as within a seed a flower is hiding, within a mantra the seeds for change – new ways of thinking, living and being – are waiting to spring forth.

A student once came to me heartbroken. His girlfriend had abruptly dropped him. After making too many phone calls to her he finally realized that he had to let go but could not. His mind gave him no rest, constantly replaying every last thing she said and everything he wished could have gone differently. He could not break the cycle. He was miserable and could not stop torturing himself with a past that could not be changed and a future never to be.

His mind was like a wild horse running back to a familiar pasture. Our thoughts are like that. They get stuck, even in unpleasant places. Just like any habit we would like to break, the mind needs to be redirected to a more powerful place of focus. A mantra is a powerful magnet even for the most runaway train of thoughts.

Mantras rewire the brain activity. Once the new pathway is established, it becomes the favored trail to travel and ultimately erases the mental wiring that no longer serves us. With the brain disengaged from a thought-life that is draining, you have a chance to put that mind to a better use. Your meditation will make your brain function better. This will support all you do with new creativity and clarity.

One of the simplest mantras to add to your basic yogic breath is "SO HUM." "SO" imitates the sound of the breath as it comes in. "HUM" is like the sigh of the exhalation as it leaves.

This ancient mantra will create equilibrium between the right and left sides of the brain and is easy to remember anytime unproductive thoughts fill your spare time. You can "chant" SO HUM soundlessly - inside your mind - thinking SO as you hear and feel the inhalation fill your heart and thinking HUM as you feel the exhalation flow out. Over time your mind will prefer to move to a happy state of balance and clarity instead of entertaining outdated conflict and confusion. You will find your mind choosing to redirect to productive life-affirming thoughts far more quickly and more often. Remember... a mantra liberates and protects your freedom of thought.

The Practice

- Practice your Basic Yogic Breath.

- Allow the breath to slow and deepen.

- Once it is effortless, add the syllable SO to your inhalation and HUM to your exhalation.

- Continue with the breath and the inner focus of SO HUM, and absorb the penetration of a spiritual alignment meeting the focus of your mind.

- Just be.

- Watch.

- Wait.

- Absorb.

- Let the mantra inhabit all of you.

- Let your Self inhabit the mantra.

- Try 54 repetitions. Work towards 108. 108 is the traditional number of beads on a strand or "Mala" used in a traditional meditation practice to count the number of repetitions. This seals the mind to a single focus and a place of power.

Sensory Meditation for Two
This creative meditation is based on the blissful experience of raising erotic energies through your sensitive touch. The purpose is not focused around the idea of turning your partner on or racing toward an orgasm. It's to observe the flow of erotic currents in your body much the way you have learned to drop into the flow of your breathing. Before you begin...

A Word to the Giving Partner:
The practice is for you.
It is not about your partner.
Touch is a portal to the present moment.
The door is open. The time is now.

You don't need to please or be pleased.
You don't have to ask what your partner wants or needs.
You don't have to perform in any way...
All you are here to do is experience...
To enter this touch as if it is the first touch you have ever given.

For now, you have no ideas about touch...
No history to say touch is good or bad...
No agenda such as "I wish to touch here or there."

You are drawn into the moment of this touch. What is it?

What is communicating to your heart through your hands?
What is this mystery, this journey, this path?
Live in this touch as it comes alive your hands.
Allow your receptivity to expand.
Where does your touch touch you back?

Feel the life force in your body penetrate the other.
Follow, one breath at a time, as your whole being awakens to this moment. Just this one.

A Word to the Receiving Partner:
The practice is for you.
It is not about your partner.
Touch is a portal to the present moment.
The door is open. The time is now.

You don't need to please or be pleased.
You don't have to say thank you.
You don't have to perform in any way.
All you are here to do is experience...
To drink in touch as if it is the first touch you have ever received it.
For now, you have no ideas about touch...
No history to say touch is good or bad...
No desire such as "I wish to be touched here or there."

You are drawn into the moment of this touch. What is it?

Allow your receptivity to expand.
Imagine inhaling and exhaling through your cells.
Feel your body become less dense.
Let sensation fill the space between each cell.
Let touch resonate where it will.
Listen to its echo with your nerve endings...
The delicate hairs on your arms...
Or the life force in your genitals.

Reach into each sensation and allow each sensation to reach into you.Flow through the rivers of energy opened with each stroke. Absorb each touch like water on sand.Let touch penetrate every layer of your awareness.

Breathe, melt, open, BE - alive to this moment. Just this one.

And for Both:
As you follow the sensations in your body, your receptivity will blossom, unfolding new petals of awareness that may extend far beyond the touch itself. A lot can happen in the extended moment of fingertips meeting thigh and thigh meeting fingertips. This is

yours to discover.

Drink deeply of the sweetness of your partner's presence, satisfying a need for nurture beyond lovemaking. Sensuality takes time to awaken.

Enjoy the awakening.

CONSCIOUS TOUCH
It all begins with a Conscious Touch. A conscious touch bears the gift of full presence. A touch with full presence communicates that there is nowhere but HERE... No other time but NOW... Nowhere else you would rather be.

This is a touch that has arrived home rather than just passing by.

A touch without hurry... complete and satisfying.
Touch - to experience the gift of touching.
Stroke - like a match draws fire.

Take the light of consciousness into your hands.
Consider each touch as an intimate conversation.

Let your hand fall like a leaf... Be there.

The Practice

Giving Partner:
To begin, sit comfortably on a bed, a soft rug or on your floor with pillows for support. Extend your right leg forward and tuck your left foot to your right inner thigh. Draw your partner's head to rest snuggly against your left thigh as it now makes a natural pillow for your partner to lean into. Your extended right leg will rest gently alongside your partner's body as another layer of support and contact.

Receiving Partner:
Assist yourself in becoming comfortable. Make yourself at home in the nest of your partner's lap. Extend both legs forward or bend both knees and plant your feet a hip width apart. In this position you can rest your inner knees together to further relax your low back.

Together:
Take some time to settle in. Sit quietly with your Basic Yogic Breath. Gradually bring your breathing into sync with your partner's.

Wait for a feeling of connection to arrive between yourself and your partner... yourself and your breathing... the breath as it extends into the space around you... and back again, filling the space that exists deep inside.

Close your eyes to deepen the calling IN of your senses. Withdraw your awareness from external clutter to focus instead on the presence of touch.

Giving Partner:
Begin with light fingertips placed upon your partner's brow. Not pressing, but light as a feather. See if you can feel a tingly buzz emanating from the point where you meet. Imagine that you can inhale and exhale through your fingertips. How does it feel? Imagine you are blind and you have only your fingertips to form an image of this divine mystery beneath your touch.

Slowly trace your partner's brow, eyelids, cheeks, lips, ears, neck, and collarbone with this delicate touch. Touch to experience touch as if it were for the first time. Open to each breath and let its current carry sensory information from fingertips to cells. Let your whole body flush with delicate warmth.

When you are ready, change your roles and practice again from the other point of view.

We chose to have our touch experience in the sensitive area of the face, neck, and ears. You could just as happily focus on the sole of one foot, the length of the spine or the nipple of one breast. The idea is to become ultra aware. Does the fingertip tracing your nipple send rushes of energy elsewhere?

As you become adept at following feeling with the body and the mind, you will be able to let pleasure overflow from cell to cell. Your whole being lights up, tingles, and hums. This is where ecstasy lives.
Yes, in you.

Chapter 6: Getting Physical Postures for Self Study

The physical practice, or the postures of yoga, makes the body flexible and strong while drawing the mind and emotions into a similar place of clarity and peace.

Releasing tension through breathing and stretching clears your body, mind and emotions of static energies, stress, mental dullness, and fatigue. Yoga can move your whole being toward relaxation and joy, all which will increase your capacity for sexual pleasure and emotional fulfillment.

The happiness of being in a body - your own - that is fully alive with vitality is a sensual and sometimes ecstatic experience. Your solo yoga practice will become a large part of the process as you learn to completely accept, nurture and cherish yourself.

As you practice yoga postures something beautiful begins to happen. Not only will your body respond to your loving care with better health and an improved physique but you may find your mind and emotions reflecting the same joyful ease. At first you may only be aware of correctly aligning knees over ankles, or getting frustrated about the elusive nature of finding balance in a standing pose. Later, as stability is achieved, the mind can go deeper, moving away from the physical activity alone to tap into the present quality of the life itself.

Each asana is an intimate invitation to become fully alive. At first we are primarily cognizant of the big muscles and joints opening. As the mind learns to move its intelligence from the constant whir of thoughts to the deeper Hum of the body, you will find that there is much that usually goes unnoticed.

As you hold your pose you may start to notice how the breath feels in this one as compared to another, how your body expands and contracts, how your skin tingles as it stretches and how a slow glow warms your muscles. The sole of your foot on the floor seems to inform the rest of you with a sense of peaceful stability while your arms stretched upward bring in freedom and energy.

We are full of deep rhythms and subtle sensations. Each focus followed returns us to the simple bliss of being.

This is an entry to that "present moment" experience people often speak of. When you become fully absorbed in a posture, the grace and strength found there penetrates every layer of your being as a whole. You are not a body in a pose; you are the experience of vitality and peace sparkling cell to cell.

The postures in this book gently cover the basic positions necessary for a good yoga practice. They will loosen your hips, ease your back and open the heart center. We have also chosen postures that work to support your endocrine system, which is responsible for the healthy hormonal balance that nourishes and rejuvenates the sex organs and keeps the body young. A regular and varied yoga practice will support the health and activity of all the organs, glands, and vital systems of the body.

Seated Postures work to open your hips, knees, and groin. The upright position of your back makes breathing easy. Engaging a full yogic breath while you hold your pose steady will calm the mind and stretch the muscles of the heart. Circulation to your whole body will increase as an additional gift.

Forward Bends add strength and flexibility to your back. They also support good adrenal function and induce relaxation as they allow your senses to turn within. Forward Bends compress the organs in the abdominal area, allowing them to relax and receive a good dose of fresh circulation.

Twists refresh the spine and work intimately with your inner body. The organs are squeezed and then flushed with blood as you hold the twist to each side. The sex organs and glands are nourished as well as the nerve centers along the spine. The hips, groin and spine will become supple and you will have more energy. Your breathing will be slow and deep.

Back Bends energize the whole body and increase blood flow through the liver and spleen. Back bending postures also lift depression and cleanse the body of fatigue.

Standing Postures support a healthy cardiovascular system while adding strength and flexibility to the major muscles and joints. They promote a focused mind and increased vigor.

Inversions assist in sending circulation to the heart, lungs and brain. We spend most of the day on our feet. Turning the world upside down with a relaxing yoga posture is a healthy change in perspective.

Supine Postures allow the body to gather the energy required for more strenuous activities like rolling around in bed with your partner. Reclined Postures have the added benefits of relaxing your body, mind, muscles and joints.

Another nice plus: yoga postures have a habit of following you off the mat! Child's Pose, for example, can return a frazzled person to sanity. As you learn to find peace on demand, peace will touch all you do. The cool collected strength of Warrior One extends itself to "grace under fire." Triangle Pose teaches multitasking as we find center while opening to all directions.

As you practice yoga you may fall more deeply in love with your own experience of life. As you find greater satisfaction in yourself, you become your own source. You need less and have more to share. From this place of personal equilibrium you can come to your relationships on full rather than empty. This is a wonderful place to be... a place where you can just breathe.

The Pranayamas, or breathing techniques you use with your postures, will guide your senses within as you learn to expand your awareness to the fullest. This heightened sense of awareness extends first to your experiencing of yourself, and later to your experiencing yourself experiencing your partner. A few languorous stretches alone is the perfect preparation for sharing a yoga practice with your partner and for the deeper harmony of making love. Let's get started...

Solo Positions

Basic Warm-Up

BACK RELEASE WITH CIRCLING

1. Sit comfortably cross legged. Place your palms on the floor in front of you. Point your fingertips inward, toward center. Your arms will form a soft circle of support.

2. As you exhale, drop into the relaxed weight of your upper body. Bend your arms. Let go of the weight of your head at the end of your spine. Lengthen each exhalation to maximize feelings of release through the back and the hips.

3. Try swaying side to side or add circles.

4. Bring your breath and movement into sync, allowing the breath to move the body.

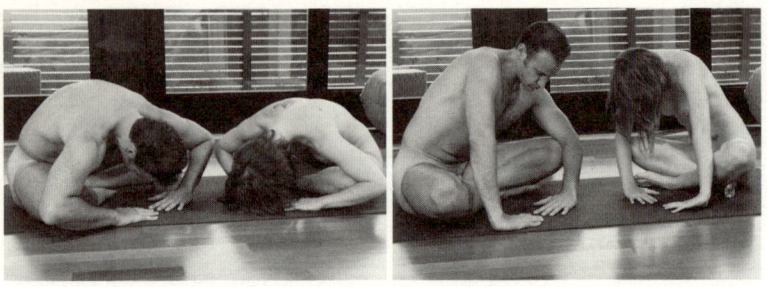

As you do this exercise, move your awareness to your lower body. Settle into your sit bones rooted to the ground. Feel the earthy quality of your relaxed buttocks, the weight of your thighs, and the softness of your palms meeting the firmness of the floor.

As you continue this exercise move your awareness upward. As you move with each breath, note how the stability of your lower body gives freedom to the upper body. Follow every sensual second of being fully alive to the energy streaming through your body. Free your upper body to ride the wave rhythm of each breath. Be like a blade of grass in the wind, a snake in the sun, a fern head unfurling.

Look for feelings of pleasure in your body. Find these moments and lean into them, awakening new layers of subtle sensation across your back and through your hips, wherever they reach.

A Back Release works with your adrenal glands and massages the kidneys. It induces relaxation and draws circulation through your sexual core.

SIMPLE TWIST WITH SIDE OPENER

1. Inhale, drawing the breath upward as if from below the body to support a long open back.

2. Exhale and twist to your right, placing your left hand on your right knee and placing your right hand behind you for support.

3. Roll your right shoulder back, opening the heart, and send your gaze in the same direction as the right shoulder.

4. Hold here for several cycles of breath. Let the breath create a deep internal massage, cleansing the organs and freeing the spine.

5. Inhale, keeping your left hand where it is on the right knee. Lift the right hand upward and slightly over to the left.

6. Draw your right bicep toward your ear and lean gently left, the left hand at your knee continuing to offer support. Breathe deeply and evenly for several cycles, allowing your side body to open and energize.

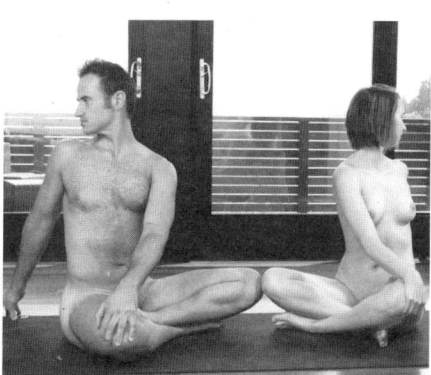
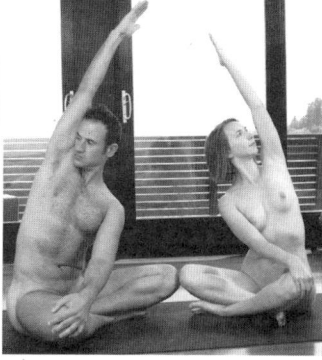

7. Return to center.

8. Repeat to the other side.

Twists rejuvenate the spine and massage the organs and glands that live in the abdominal area. Deep twists held for 7-10 yogic breaths will tone the organs by assisting in detoxification of the organs.

Side Openers in general help to create more room for you to breathe and for the organs there to function with ease. Our organs become compressed as our upper body responds to a lifetime of gravity and "shrink."

Breathe into those inner spaces. Open up. Feel your body come alive with fresh life force.

This supports adrenal function.

HIP RELEASE
1. From seated, bend your left leg at the knee and plant your heel close to your sit bones.

2. Draw your right knee in toward your chest. Rest the outer edge of your right foot or ankle comfortably on your left thigh. Your right knee will be angled outward, toward your right side.

3. Place your hands on the floor behind you. Relax. Focus on gently unwinding the tension from your right hip, one breath at a time. Hold for several cycles of breath.

4. Repeat on the other side.

You can make this deeper by moving your hips closer to your heel and your hands closer to your hips on the floor behind you. This pulls the upper body upright and tight against the thigh of the side you are working with. You will feel stronger releases through your hip. Go slowly to prevent over stretching. Loose hips are fun. Torn muscles are not.

This posture supports healthy sexual function as it both relaxes and nourishes the sex organs and glands.

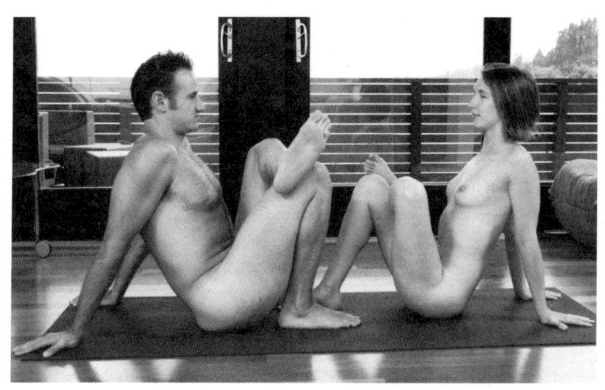

HEAD ROLLS
1. Exhale, relaxing your chin down toward your chest.

2. Inhale, slowly rolling your head toward your right shoulder.

3. Exhale and relax into the weight of your head, counter-balanced by the relaxed weight of your left shoulder.

4. Pause for 5 cycles of breath, feeling the length of your neck and trapezium open as tensions dissipate and harmony is restored.

5. Repeat all to the other side.

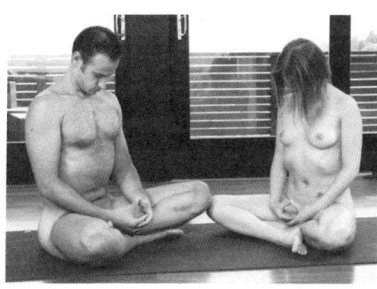 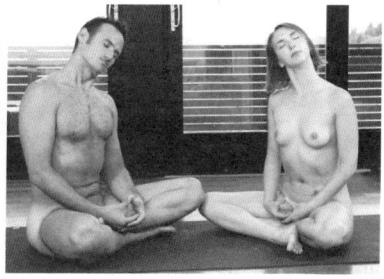

This practice relieves tension from the neck and works with the thyroid gland.

ENERGIZING BREATH
1. From seated: bring both hands forward and interlace your fingers. Place your hands on the back of your head and drop your

chin toward your chest. Pause here for a few cycles of breath.

2. Draw your awareness within, following the breath as it travels from deep in the base of your belly upward, lengthening your spine and sending your chest to meet your chin. Exhale, allowing all tension to fall away from your neck, shoulders and back.

3. With the next inhalation, draw the breath in and up. Stretch your spine up and away from your hips, lifting your head, pressing the back of your head into the support of your hands while opening your elbows out side to side.

4. Exhale and return your chin to your chest, elbows relaxed, head heavy at the end of your spine. Your upper body remains upright. Do not slouch forward or round your back.

5. Repeat several times. Bring the breath and body into union. Be slow and unhurried.

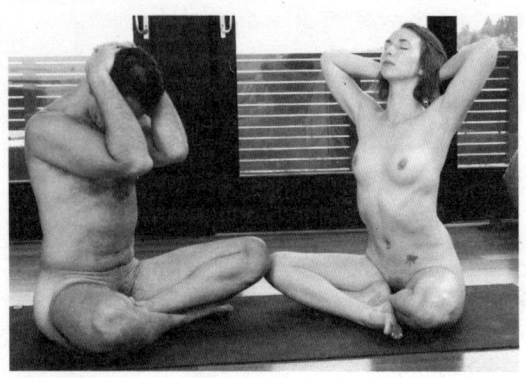

CAT STRETCHES
1. Move to Table Pose, on all fours. Place your hands shoulder width apart and your knees hip width apart.

2. Inhale. Lead with the tip of your tail bone, tilting it upward while making a deep valley of your back, flexing your spine and lifting your gaze upward.

3. Exhale. Draw your tailbone under while rounding the back. Drop your head at the end of your spine and send your gaze

toward your navel.

You can make this stronger by pulling your navel inward toward your spine during the exhalation. This will tone your abdomen, empty your lungs of stale air and give your internal organs a friendly squeeze. This sensual, playful pose releases tension throughout the whole mind/body system and keeps your spine young. All that, and it feels so good too.

4. Continue to flow with the present movement of each breath. Bring the breath and body together as one. Find moments of effortlessness. Move for the sheer pleasure of moving.

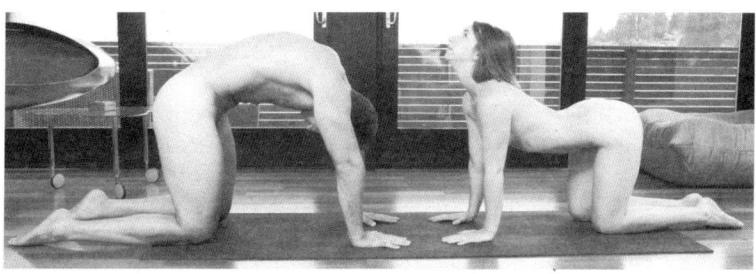

Be water, be wave, be mountaintop, be valley.
Find your inner animal. Purr.

MODIFIED CAMEL POSE
Back bending postures are energizing and great to cleanse stress-related fatigue from your body/mind.

1. Kneel with knees a hip width apart.

2. Roll your shoulders up toward your ears and then down your back toward your hips. This opens the heart center and wraps your shoulder blades into place on your

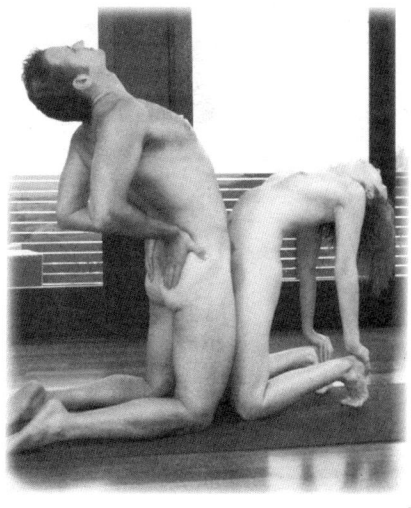

back.

3. Move your thighs and hips forward. Inhale, lifting upward through your heart center.

4. Exhale, rolling your shoulders down and away from your ears.

5. Take several cycles of breath here. Feel the gentle crescent shape of your body, opening the heart and energizing the spine.

All back bends stimulate the central nervous system and help your body cope with stress.

Backbends are a natural restorative for nervous exhaustion and depression, and support liver and spleen function.

PUPPY DOG STRETCH
1. From kneeling, bend forward and return to Table Pose.

2. Walk your hands forward until your back is open to its full length, lowering your head and chest to the ground while keeping your hips high, aligned over your knees.

3. Stay here for several cycles of breath, letting your heart open and your back release.

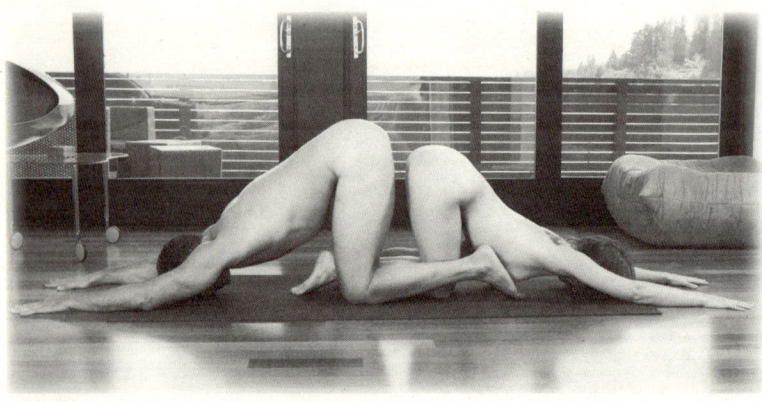

Forward Bends encourage relaxation and reduce stress.

This posture relaxes the heart, opens your shoulders and frees the spine from fatigue. It also draws awareness and circulation through the perineum.

WIDE LEGGED FORWARD BEND

1. Step your feet side to side in a standing straddle position about four feet apart.

2. Hinge forward from your hips. Place your palms on the floor a shoulder width apart.

3. Bend at the elbows to gradually lower your head toward the floor.

4. Glide your hands down the outsides of your legs to grasp the outer edges of your feet.

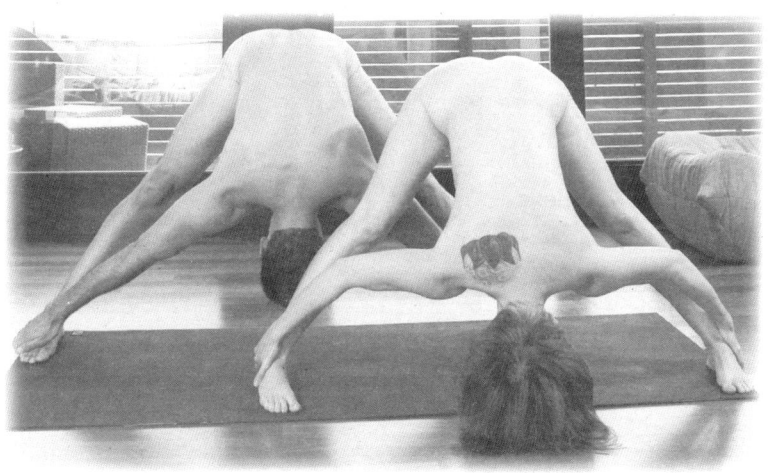

If you cannot comfortably reach your feet, plant your palms to the floor and walk them backward, in between your feet, as far as you can - easing your way into this Forward Bend.

5. Exhale into the relaxed weight of your body. Drop the weight of your head at the end of your spine.

6. Feel your spine lengthen as you reverse the effects of gravity one breath at a time.

Your hips, thighs and groin will also thank you.

As a Forward Bend, this posture is a natural stress buster.

It also reverses the effects of age and gravity by decompressing the discs between the vertebrae.

The perineum, sex glands and organs receive vital circulation in this posture.

WARRIOR TWO

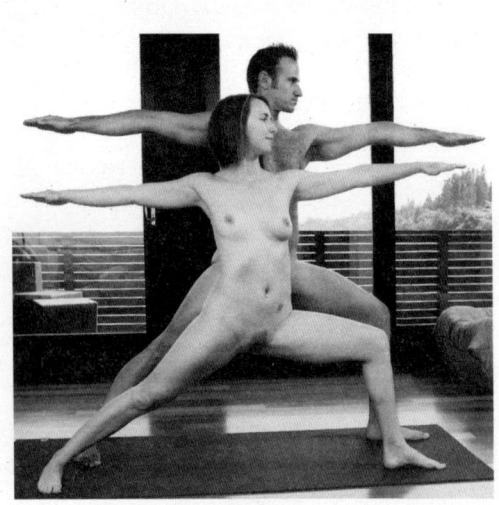

1. Step your feet side to side in a standing straddle position about 4 feet apart. Pivot on your right heel and point your toes.

2. Press your left heel slightly back, placing that foot on a gentle diagonal angle. Draw your hips under your shoulders.

3. Center your head over your heart. Lift each arm out to your sides at shoulder level. Send your gaze over the fingertips of the right hand.

4. Feel your feet on the floor. Feel your hips and heart open to the sides.

5. Feel the peaceful strength resident in this posture. Just be here, strong and steady, the breath smooth and even.

6. After several cycles of breath, repeat to your other side.

This posture aligns the chakras along the length of the spine. It is a natural hip and heart opener, and adds strength to your legs, back and shoulders.

TRIANGLE

1. From Warrior Two, straighten your left leg with your hands, hips and heart still wide open to the side.

2. Press your right hip out, lifting your right hand to vertical. Simultaneously reach your left hand down to below your knee.

3. Anchor your back foot. Feel your side open and spine lengthen.

4. Send your lower ribs slightly forward while relaxing gently back into your upper ribs. Extend energy and awareness though the length of both arms.

5. Rest firmly into the support of your feet on the floor. Allow energies to unwind from deep center - freeing the sacral area, the hips, and the heart.

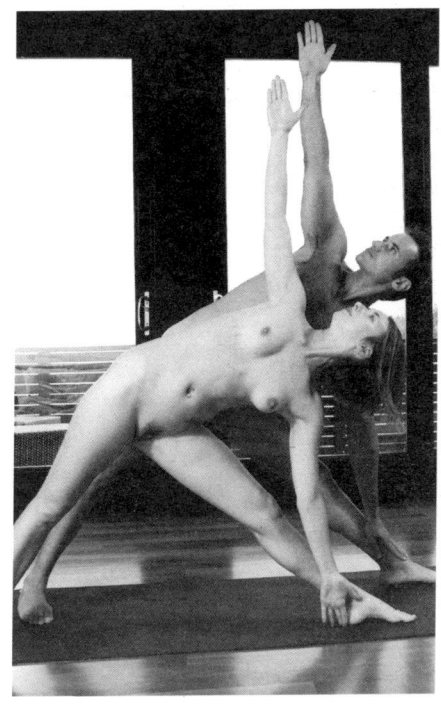

6. Repeat to the other side.

Triangle works with the energies of the Root, Sacral and Heart Chakras. It is both grounded and liberating, as the wide foundation of the feet allows for a dynamic reach in multiple directions.

Breathe deeply and follow the sensations in your body. Note your "wingspan" from the fingertips of one hand to the other. Expand from your heart in all four directions - up, down, front and back.

Breathe with your whole body.

EAGLE POSE

1. From standing, place your feet a hip width apart. Softly bend your knees.

2. Draw your right thigh to rest across your left thigh. You can bring your hands out, side to side at shoulder level, to assist with balance if you need.

3. Place your hands together, palm to palm as if in prayer.

4. (For Modified Eagle) Bend your knees a little more deeply. Bring your head and heart slightly forward of your hips, keeping your spine long.

5. Try wrapping your foot around your calf. Rest into the power of your legs twined together.

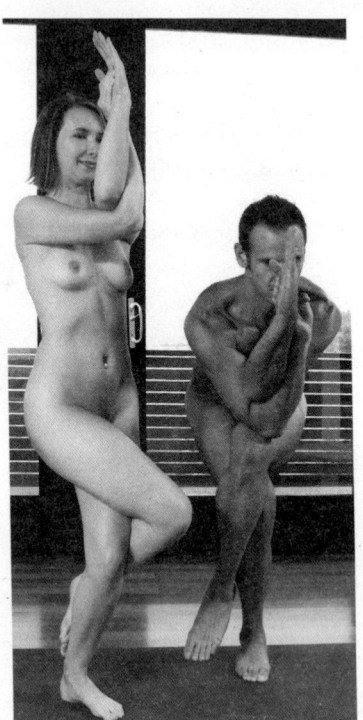

6. Wrap your left arm under your right. Gently squeeze your arms and legs together, drawing your energies and circulation back from your extremities, toward your vital organs and sexual core.

7. (For Full Eagle) Quiet your mind as you focus on each breath, holding this posture with a combination of rootedness, strength and balance.

DOWNWARD FACING DOG

1. Return to Table Pose, onto all fours. Flex your feet and tuck your toes under.

2. Rolling up onto the balls of your feet, gradually lift your hips and heels high.

3. Exhale as you send your hips and thighs back, your heels dropping toward the floor. Press forward into your hands, opening your back to its fullest length.

4. A soft bend to your knees is fine. Straighten your legs if you can, without overstretching your hamstrings.

5. Move your shoulders away from your ears, relaxing your head at the end of your spine.

6. Hold for several cycles of breath.

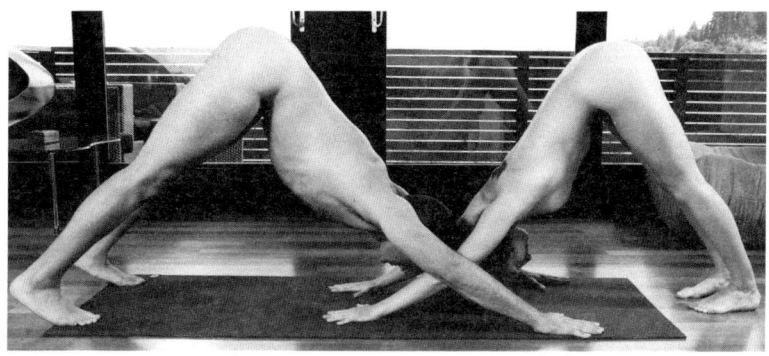

This posture stretches out the whole back of your body, from your hands up to your hips, and from your hips down to your heels. Follow the flow of sensation from the relaxed weight of your head at the end of the spine all the way up to the tip of your tailbone. Lift the perineum up slightly and press back through your thighs.

This is stimulating for the sex glands and relaxes the heart. Imagine breathing into your kidneys as your upper body becomes buoyant with each inhalation. Let the heart descend a little with each exhalation, resting.

Imagine that your spine is a hollow reed. Imagine the breath clearing the chakras as it flows in and out - as if moving up and down inside the length of your spine. Imagine each breath piercing the center of each chakra as it rises and falls. Tune into what you feel.

PIGEON POSE
1. Start in Downward Facing Dog.

2. Bend your left knee and draw it forward beneath your body.

3. Shift your weight onto both hands, plant your knee near the thumb of your right hand, while your right heel finds its place near your left hip.

4. Now glide back through the length of your left leg, straightening it out as you lower your hips to or toward the floor.

5. If your hips are stiff and finding the floor is difficult, slide a firm pillow or folded blanket under your left sit bone and rest into its support. Or you can imitate the posture pictured on the left. This posture offers the same benefits but the intensity of the stretch is completely in your hands.

6. Hold for several cycles of breath, unwinding the hips and energizing the area around the Root Chakra, the groin and sexual centers.

7. Step back to Downward Facing Dog.

8. Repeat, bending the other leg.

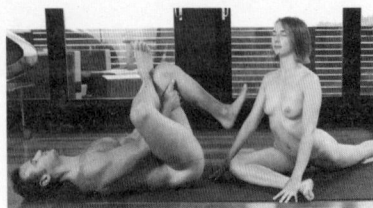 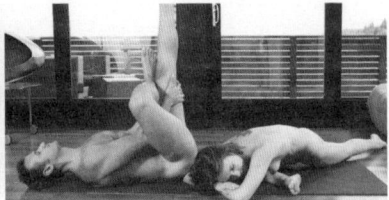

KNEES TO CHEST POSE
1. Lie down on your back. Bend both knees and pull them into your chest.

2. Wrap both arms around the knees and clasp your hands together, encircling your knees within the embrace of your arms.

3. You can deepen your pose by allowing your knees to move outward in the direction of your ribs or even slightly past them to each side.

4. Now breathe fully and deeply into the whole body. Feel yourself expand with each inhalation and return to center with each exhalation.

5. Let all tension drain away. Hold here for several cycles of breath, returning to a place of perfect support and deep peace.

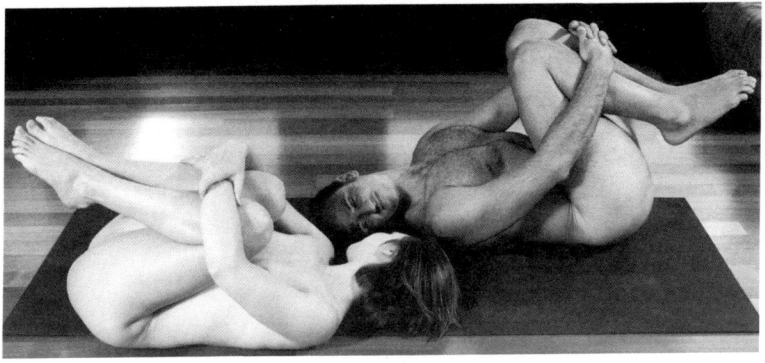

This relaxes your back, hips and sex organs.

PLOW POSE
1. From Knees to Chest Pose, release your arms from your knees and straighten your legs.

2. Visualize pressing the soles of your feet onto the ceiling and your thighs away, as if pressing them against an imaginary wall.

3. From here, press your palms down to the floor on either side of your hips, slowly sending your feet backward in the direction of your head.

4. As your hips lift off the floor, place your hands at your lower back for support. Continue to relax your toes toward the floor just behind your head.

5. Your weight should be falling through your hips into your hands and across the back of your heart area, up to the tops of your shoulders.

6. Your chin and chest will move toward one another. If your feet do not reach the floor, just let them hover wherever they are.

7. Be sure to keep the weight of your hips away from your neck, resting instead back and into your hands. Breathe smoothly and

evenly for several cycles.

Plow Pose promotes flexibility of the spine and releases tension in the pelvis. As your chin and chest move together, this posture stimulates your thyroid, parathyroid, and pineal glands. Your heart, brain and lungs are also nourished as the posture directs the flow of blood to these vital organs.

Use your Ujjayi Breathing here to work more deeply with the thyroid. Draw your awareness to the cool sensation of the breath flowing through the cave of the throat center. Listen to the sound. Follow the rise of your energies as they seem to move in the direction of your crown as Plow Pose helps to clear the upper chakras.

8. Roll down one vertebra at a time.

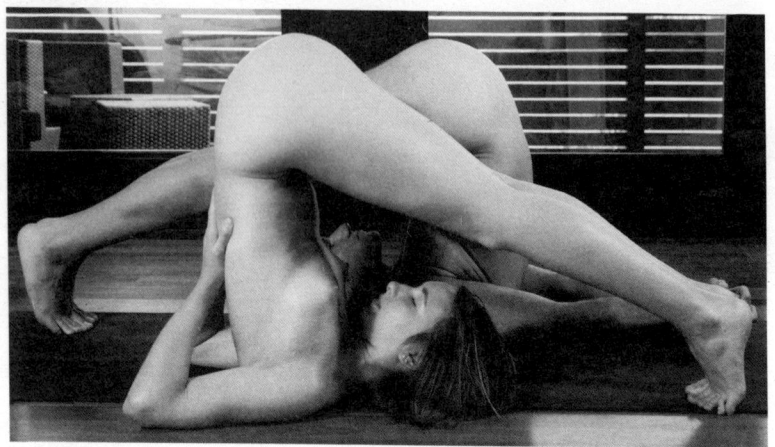

9. Relax again in Knees to Chest Pose.

SUPINE ANGLE POSE
1. From Knees to Chest Pose, straighten your legs as you did when moving to Plow Pose.

2. Relax your legs out to each side, making a supine straddled stance.

3. You can assist yourself to a deeper posture by resting your hands on your inner thighs, calves, or feet while gently but firmly pulling downward.

4. Draw down and out to the sides quite firmly for a stronger assist and deeper release.

Supine Angle Pose relaxes the vaginal wall muscles and helps restore energy to the genitals.

5. Hold for several cycles of breath.

6. Return to Knees to Chest Pose.

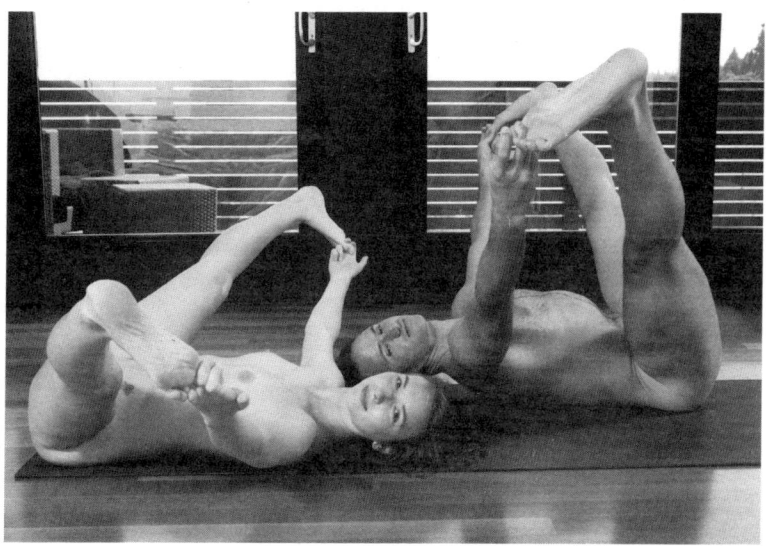

CORPSE POSE
1. Stretch both legs forward and down. Roll your palms skyward at either side of the hips, opening the heart and relaxing the shoulders.

2. Exhale, settling into the support of the earth below the body. Inhale, opening into the lightness of space inside and all around you.

Enjoy a completely relaxed and revitalized you!

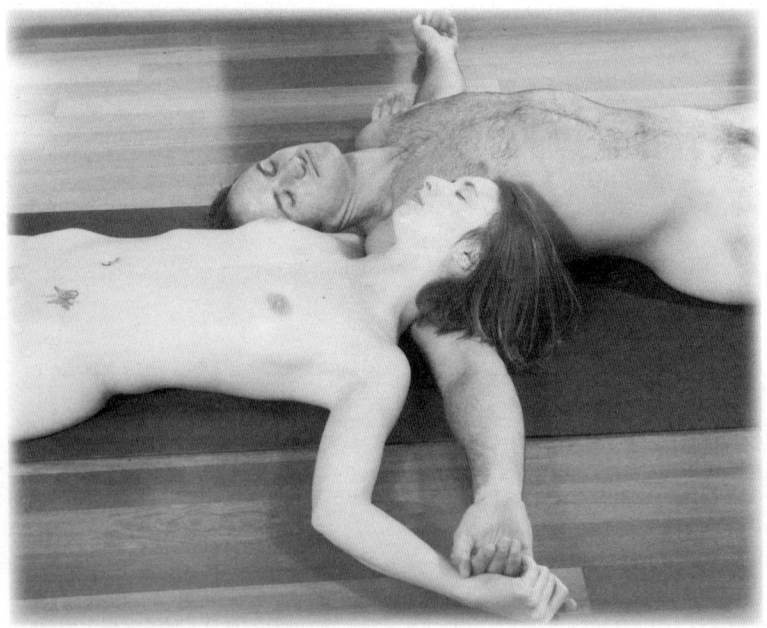

Chapter 7: Partnered Postures
Building Touch and Energy

The postures in this chapter are fun. They bring you together in new and interesting ways. Partner
postures extend an invitation to intimacy.

Many of the postures reflect the joy and energy of lovemaking while some forge new bonds in the
areas of trust. All of the postures share a balance of strength and power, peace and depth, bringing
your body/mind to a place of restored well-being and increased vitality.

You may have fallen head over heels in love with each other, but when was the last time you were
feet over head together? As you move from pose to pose you find new ways to hold one another
while the challenges to your strength and balance make a perfect reflection of what it takes to stay
in a loving relationship. Splits, anyone?

The practices you share today will have positive effects that ripple outward from the heart to connect with all you do in subtle ways that create profound shifts - shifts towards more joy, more freedom, more
honesty, more communication, deeper intimacy, and a sex life that is growing as much as you are.

For the yoga purist, you will find that the postures held together magnify the benefit. As a form of
exercise, nothing beats partner yoga for stress relief as you unwind together into the arms of shared stretches and postures that beg for more.

As a form of foreplay, the obvious invitation for seductive touches and deep penetration in some of
the positions is enough to ignite that inner fire.

As a whole, your partner yoga sessions build a new language between you... a vocabulary of touch and energy that will quickly become all your own. Take each posture slowly. Find your own way into its expression.

Every couple is a unique pairing. Most of you will be different sizes and shapes, weights and heights. The ideal alignments expressed by our pictures may not be how you look in the pose, so remember that the most important thing is how you feel.

Reach for the feeling and everything else will follow.

EXERCISE KEY ◙ ○ •
◙ **means working in unison**
○ **means SHE moves**
• **means HE moves**

SEATED TWIST
◙ Sit cross-legged face to face.

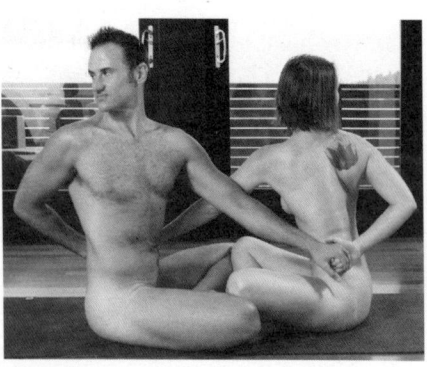

◙ Bring your right hand behind your back and as far toward your left hip as you can. Now reach with your left hand to find your partner's right hand as tucked behind his back.

◙ Keep your grip firm and sit up, keeping your spine long and lifting. Inhale drawing your awareness upward through the length of your spines. Exhale and twist in the direction of your right shoulder. Hold for 3-5 cycles of breath.

Add a Side Opener:
◙ From where you are, release your left hand and let it come to rest on your partner's upper thigh. Take your right hand from behind your back and stretch up and over toward center, meeting your partner palm to palm - and perhaps with a kiss cheek to cheek.

Pause for 3-5 cycles of breath. Absorb the energy of the pose. As you exhale, feel the rootedness of your lower body.

As you inhale, follow the lifting feeling of life force flowing upward with your focus.

As you feel your waists lengthen and your ribs expand, the posture encourages circulation to flow, supporting the kidneys and adrenal glands.

Repeat to other side.

DOUBLE JANU SIRSANA
- Sit side by side with your legs extended in front of you.

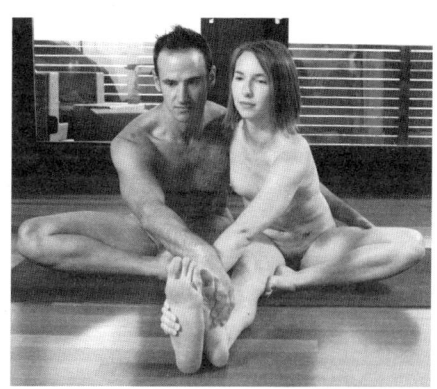

- Bend your outside leg at the knee and place your foot firmly against your upper inner thigh. Wrap your inside arms around each other's low back.

- Begin to lean forward. Reach towards your partner's extended foot as you draw your nose towards your knee.

Beginners - Reach as far forward as you can. Let your hand make supportive contact anywhere it will on the length of your leg.

Advancing - Find each other's hands and take hold of them where they can clasp around the soles of your feet.

- Pause for several cycles of breath. Feel the wave force of the breath causing your bodies to gently rise and fall. Settle into the pose one exhalation at a time.

This opens your hips and takes tension from the long muscles of your legs. Circulation and awareness are moved through the sex organs and up the length of the spine. Turn and repeat to the other side.

ASSISTED BADDHA KONASANA
- Sit face to face.

○ Move into Baddha Konasana / Bound Angle Pose by bending both legs and pressing the soles of your feet together. Keep your back long and spine straight. Relax the weight of your knees out to the sides. Reach for your partner's hands to stabilize your upper body as you allow your heels to move further toward your groin.

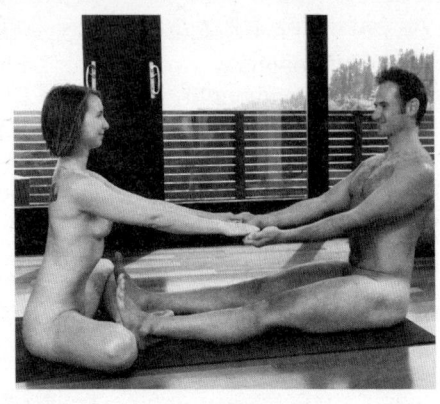

• Place your feet just above her ankles or at mid-shin while taking hold of her hands to support her upper body. Straighten your legs, sending her heels towards her sit bones. Move slowly without force. Ask her to tell you when she is getting just the right amount of stretch, support and pleasure from the pose.

Advanced variation: Add a Forward Bend.
• Draw her forward, encouraging length through her spine. Maintain gentle but firm pressure with your feet against her shins to keep her heels tucked up against her groin as she leans forward. Apply nice massage-style strokes to her back, arms, and neck. You too can lean forward and allow your weight and warmth to further assist her forward bend as you rest on her back.

○ Try reaching all the way forward to hold his thighs, hips, or even his low back.

This posture makes for flexible hips and encourages circulation to the sex organs and glands. The relaxed weight of the lower body brings our awareness to the root chakra, bringing up feelings of stability and calm.

DOUBLE CHILD'S POSE
◉ Begin from kneeling face to face. Rest your hands on your partner's shoulders.

Lean your heads forward until they touch, while moving away from each other on your knees. At the same time glide your hands from

your partner's shoulders as far down their back as you can.
Keep your palms warmly on your partner's back as you lower your
hips to rest on your heels, entering Child's Pose individually and
as one.

◉ As you settle in, separate your knees a bit to make more room
for your chest and abdomen to descend. Allow your forehead to
rest on the floor.

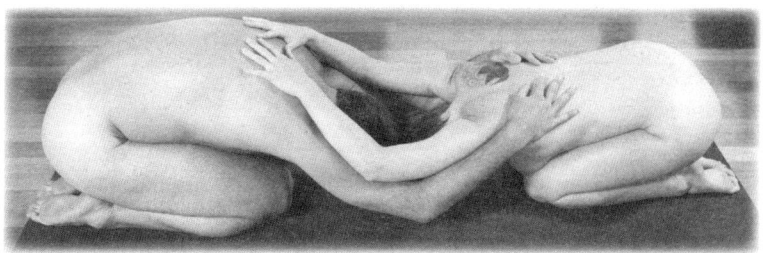

Hold in this relaxing posture for as long as you wish. Sink into the
perfect support of the Earth below you and your partner with you.

This pose tames tension in the hips and low back. It relaxes the
sex organs and nourishes the glands. The shoulders benefit from
an opening stretch as the heart center or chest is encouraged to
descend and relax.

EXTENDED CHILD'S POSE / UPWARD FACING DOG
- Stay relaxed in Child's Pose.

○ Come up to standing. Place your palms firmly to his lower back
near the sacrum. Walk your feet backward until your back is at
its fullest length. Plant your feet to the ground a hip width apart.
Press your thighs back and anchor your heels - OR - keep your
knees slightly bent if your hamstrings are tight.

Now send your weight forward into your hands. Lower your hips
and thighs and lift upward with your heart and head as you flow to
Upward Facing Dog.

Rock forward and back to repeat the shift of your weight from
hands to feet, as expressed in Upward Facing Dog and Downward
Facing Dog, several times in smooth steady motion.

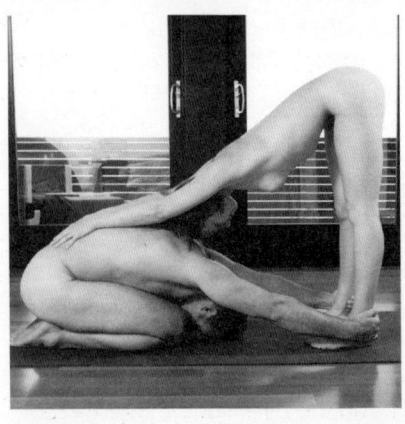 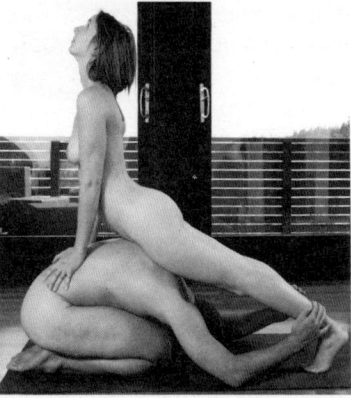

This has the delicious effect of invigorating the active partner and fully releasing tensions held in the sacrum, back and hips of the recipient.

You won't want to forget this one.

When you finish, assist ● to seated. Exchange roles and repeat with ○ receiving.

DOUBLE CAT STRETCHES
○ Move forward onto your hands and knees into Table Pose.

● Kneel behind her and press the fronts of your thighs and hips to her backside for stability. Rest your hands on her low back.

○ Begin to flex and arch your back in long fluid movements. Inhale as you flex your spine.

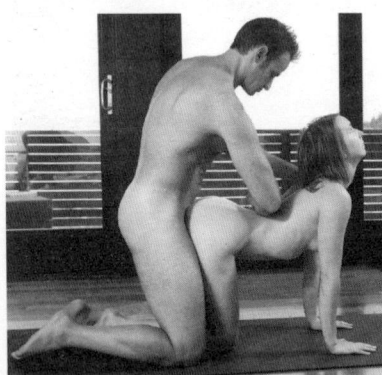 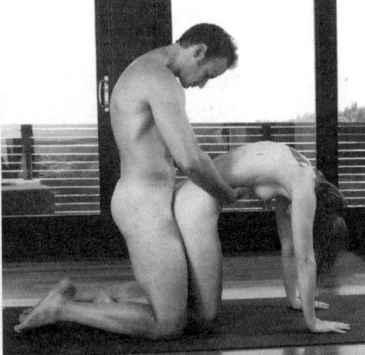

Exhale as you round your back.

• Lean into her low back with your palms or forearms as she flexes and pull up and back with your hands around her waist as she rounds her back.

◉ Fall into sync with each other, both breath and movement falling into a sensual wave of pleasurable release.

This shared posture invites playful sensuality while refreshing the length of the spine and generating a positive flow of life force and awareness from the perineum through the direction of your gaze.

Repeat for the other partner.

DOUBLE CAMEL POSE

◉ Move to kneeling with one partner in front of the other, ○ in front of ●.

• Press right up behind her. Make the posture snug.

• Wrap your hands around the sides of her hips.

○ Reach back and hold the outside of his hips or thighs with your hands.

○ Together, send your hips and thighs forward while arching back.

• Send your hips, thighs and chest into her back as support. Do not over flex your spine, just enough to create some nice movement in her direction.

○ As your hips move forward you have the luxury of leaning back into his support.

Hold for a few cycles of breath and then release into a shared hug. Repeat this swaying motion for 5 cycles before exchanging roles.

You can advance the posture by having partner ● reach his hands back to hold his heels, deeply arching his back.

From this deeper position, ○ receives far more support to open into a deeper backbend as well.

This movement juices up the spine and creates a strong feeling of mutual support and sensual energy.

DOUBLE PUPPY DOG STRETCH
From the same kneeling front to back position, ○ keeps her thighs pressed firmly against her partner while walking her hands all the way forward until her chest and chin are resting on the floor.

● Hold onto her hips as she moves forward, keeping her hips aligned directly over her knees. When she is in position, apply all kinds of loving massage strokes and squeezes. Let your hands

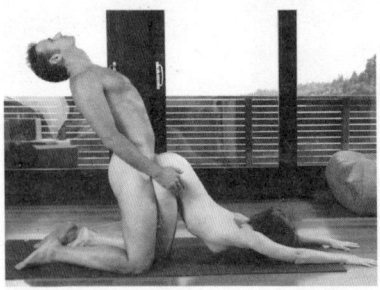 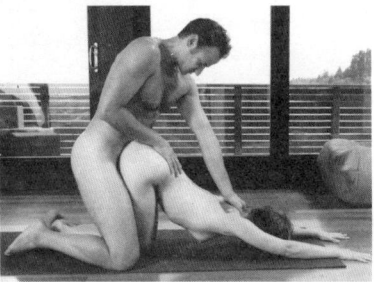

travel from hips to shoulders and back. Take your time...
Repeat the last two postures for the other partner.

This pose is an invitation for sexual play - now or later or both. The pose draws energy and awareness to the perineum, charges the sex organs and send waves of pleasure through the spine.

DOUBLE DOWNWARD FACING DOG
○ With your partner already positioned in Downward Facing Dog, place your hand on his low back and press down to encourage grounding your partner's weight back into his heels.

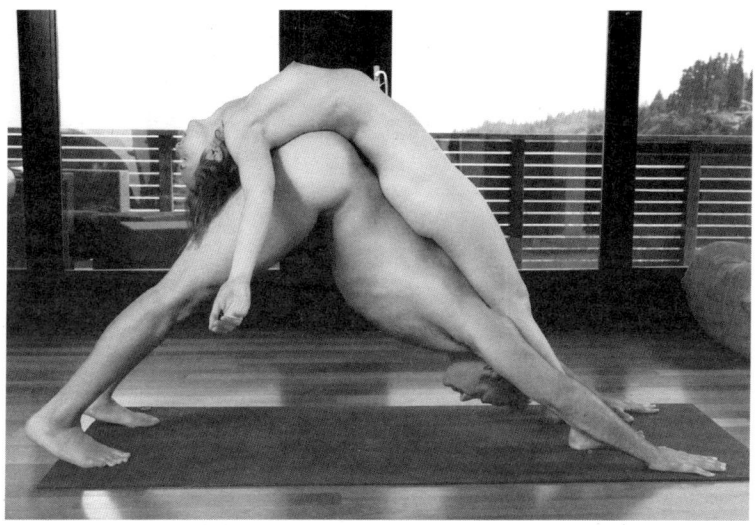

Walk around to where his hands are planted on the floor.
Step in between his hands and lay your back along the length of his, with your head and shoulders resting across his low back and hips.

In this posture, your weight is not a burden to bear but is a gift.

As you lean back and into his hips, a delightful traction occurs through the length of the spine, releasing tension. Rather than being heavy you are actually taking the pressure off of his hands and shoulders, as your presence sends his weight back and away from his hands to anchor down through his legs and feet.

You have the bliss of being supported in a perfect Heart Opener. Embrace the moment you share. It is so nice to have someone to lean on.

This pose is a great example of two distinctly different experiences coming together in perfect mutual support.

PARTNERED WIDE-LEGGED FORWARD BEND
WITH MASSAGE

○ Stand with your feet 3-4 feet apart. Fold forward from the hips bringing your head to or toward the floor. Hold here for several cycles of breath. Let go of the weight of your head. Feel your spine open, becoming longer as the effects of gravity are reversed.

You can advance the posture by reaching your hands around your legs or through the center of your feet to wrap around his legs or ankles as he is standing behind you.

● Hold her hips as she bends forward, offering stability as she lets go into the flow of gravity spilling through her back.

Apply any and all massage style strokes, or gently pummel her back with the soft side of your fists or heels of your hands.

It all feels wonderful.

The posture promotes shared

stability and relaxation. It is revitalizing for the mind and body.

This opens the whole back body, especially the buttocks, back, and hamstrings.

WARRIOR TWO

◙ Stand front to back, one assisting the other.

○ Stand as before with feet 3-4 feet apart.

◙ Turn your right foot so that your toes are pointing right. Stretch your arms out to the sides at shoulder level, facing the direction of your right forward foot. Bend the forward knee until it moves into position above the ankle. Keep your upper body aligned, head over heart and hips under shoulders.

This pose is steady, calm and focused, encouraging a harmonious balance of power, peace and strength.

- Apply supportive contact and experimental stretching.

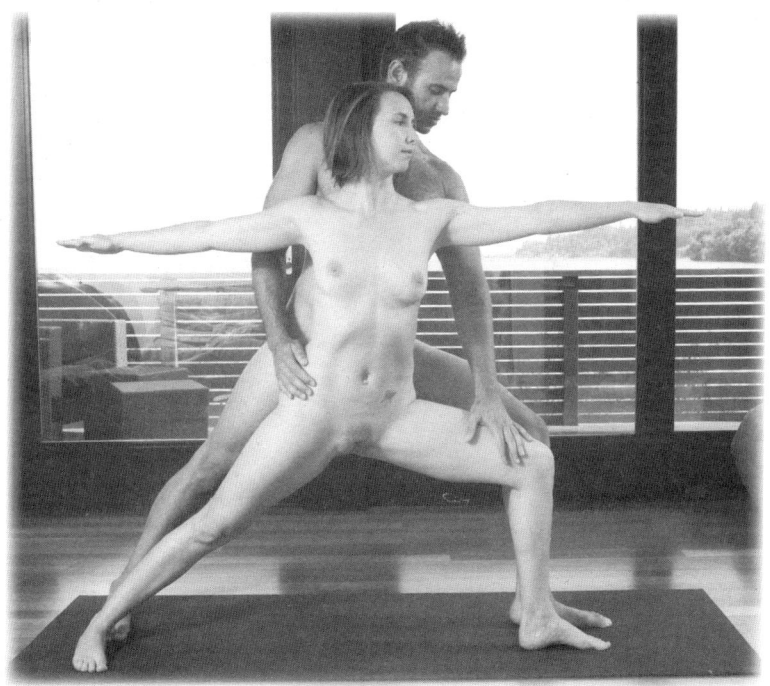

Repeat the posture to the other side and for the other partner. Treat your partner as if you are the sculptor and they are the work of art. Define each limb with your hands. Trace the length of the spine. Support the weight of the head, turning the gaze forward. Press down on the tops of the feet. Wring out the thighs with gentle squeezing.

Have fun as you open up rivers of life force to flow freely through your partner's form.

DOUBLE TRIANGLE POSE
◉ Stand front to back with your feet 3-4 feet apart. Turn the toes of your right foot to point right. Press the back heel back an inch or so, leaving that foot on a diagonal angle. Keep your legs straight and align your upper bodies - back to belly - as one.

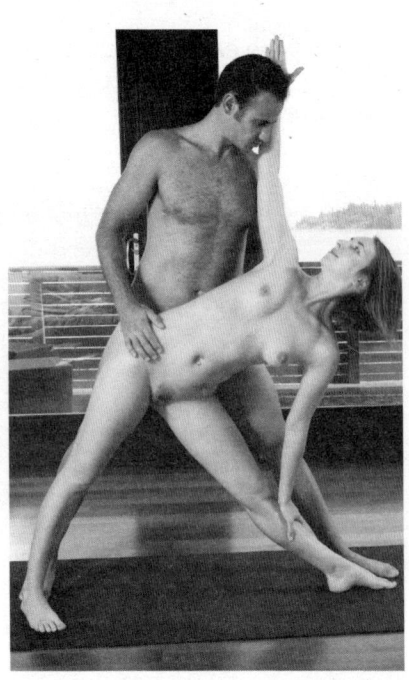

○ Move your arms out to the sides at shoulder level. Glide the forward hand down the length of your forward leg. Let your back arm lift until vertical. Turn your gaze up to meet your partner's. Keep steady contact with your arms. Press your palms to each other wherever they meet on the length of the arm.

● Treat your partner to the same support and sculpting exercise applied in Warrior Two.

In this posture it is most helpful to support the forward rotation of the lower ribs and the backward resting of the upper hip.

This is done with gentle guidance from your hands in a push me/pull you motion from behind.

Roll your partner's upper body to rest securely into your support for maximum benefits.

Continue your happy exploration.

This pose invigorates your whole system. It moves energy through all seven chakras and extends its reach in all four directions.

Triangle pose encourages vitality and balance.

FULL SAIL
◉ Stand front to back.

• Turn sideways and step your feet a full 3-4 feet apart, making a wide base of support. Take hold of her hands and rotate her arms so that her palms face outward, away from her body, with the thumbs extended upward toward the ceiling. This is an important point as this assures freedom throughthe shoulders and chest.

○ When your partner tells you he is steady, release all of your weight forward. Relax through your hips and thighs. Lift your heart and let your head fall back. Let your body open like a full sail with the wind at its back. Breathe....expand...be... Return your hips over your heels to standing upright when you are ready.

○ Keeping hold of your partner's hands, fold forward, moving in the opposite direction as your nose moves toward your knees.

This pose and counter pose open both the front and back of the body, sending life force and awareness throughout.

This is a divine trust-building exercise, as the supporting partner must be the rock for the partner daring to trust - reaching past her own center of balance and into the liberating fullness of a heart secure enough to open completely.

Repeat for the other partner.

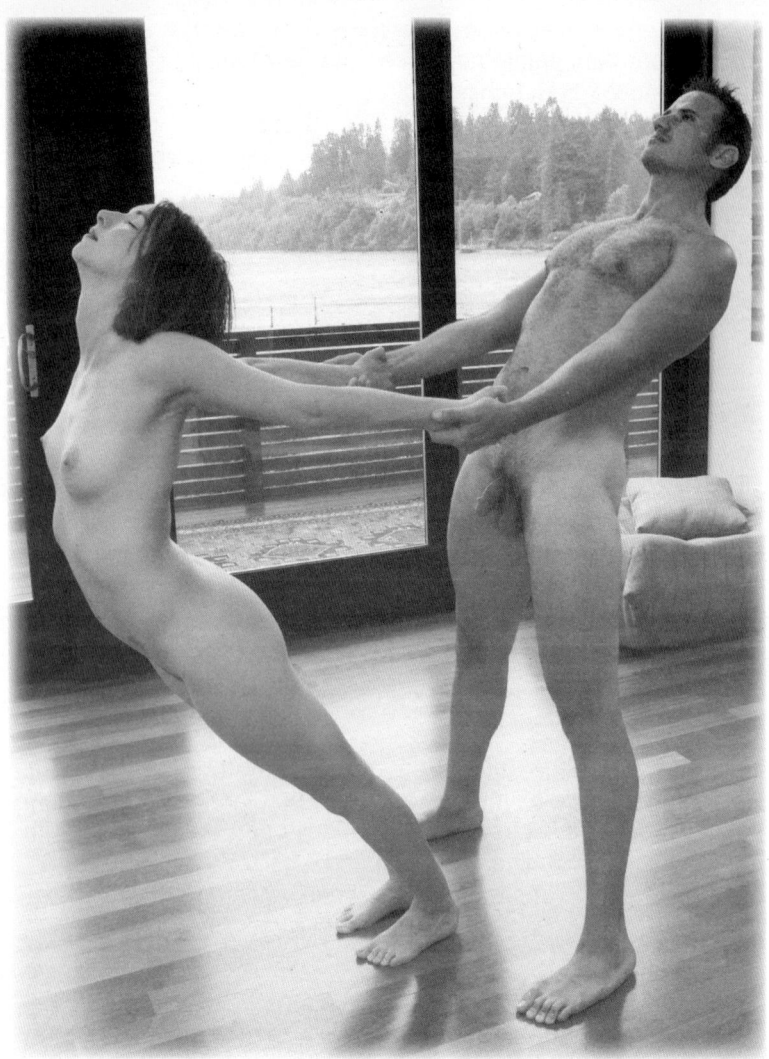

REACHING POSE
◉ Turn face to face. Place your hands on your partner's shoulders. Lean toward one another while you walk your feet backward until your hips align over your shoulders and your backs are long and open.

Your hands will glide in the direction of your partner's hips, coming to rest where they will on each other's back.

Hold here for several breaths. Feel the gentle rise and fall that

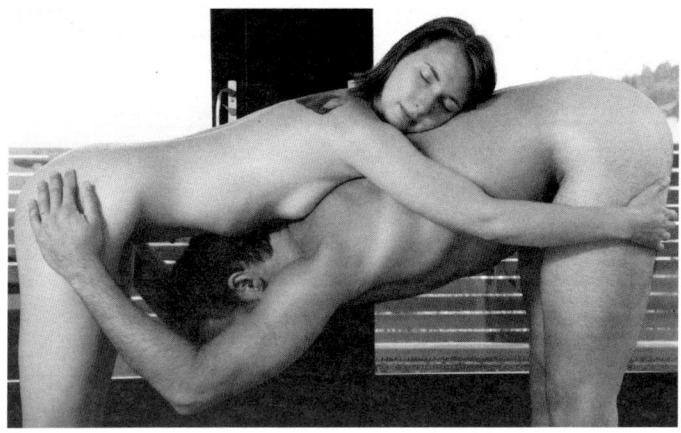

moves you with each inhalation and exhalation.
This posture uses perfect mutual support to completely open the heart, free the back and shoulders, and establish a firm foundation of caring support.

DOUBLE SQUAT
◉ From Reaching Pose, bend your knees and lower your hips toward your heels. Your hands will glide down the length of the arms to clasp firmly just above the wrist.

This is wonderful as the mutual support allows complete release for the hips, groin and low back... the circulation to the sex organs

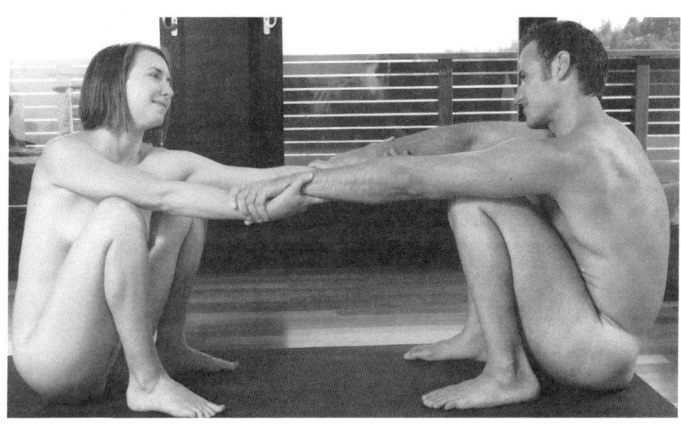

and glands a plus.

Play with the sharing of weight rocking front and back. It is all good…

DOUBLE PASCIMOTTANA-SANA / FORWARD BEND

◉ Sit facing one another with your legs extended toward your partner's hips. Reach for each other. Hold hands to start with, gradually folding forward.

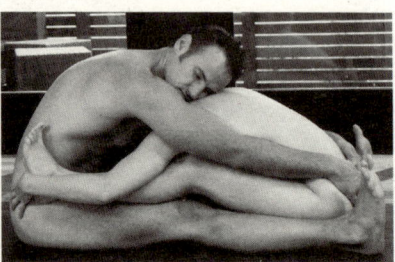

As you deepen the pose, have one partner be under and the other over, as you fold one inside the other in layers of peaceful warmth.

This pose opens the whole back of the body, working to make a flexible spine, an open low back and long hamstrings. The forward bend of the upper body massages and clears the organs housed in the abdominal cavity.

This is especially good for your adrenal glands. As tension leaves the body you will feel both relaxed and energized.

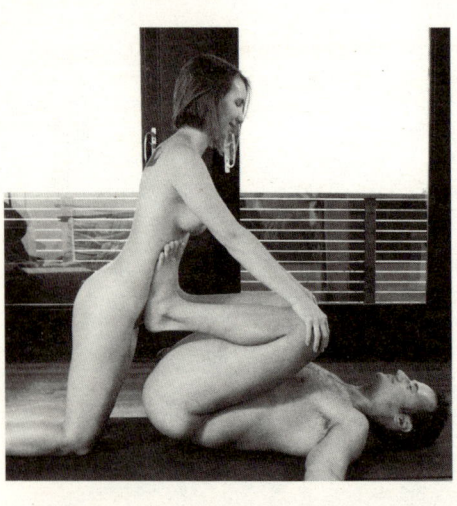

KNEES TO CHEST POSE

○ Help your partner lay down with his back on the floor.

○ Place the soles of his feet against your abdomen or at the front of each shoulder. Once contact is established, lean forward. Enjoy the support of his body as he receives the joys of your weight melting into his body.

- Let your knees fall out to the sides in the direction of your ribs. Be receptive and passive. Let go.

◉ Breathe, melt, rock side to side, release, and follow the exhaled breath into surrender. Enjoy.

The posture is an invitation to lovemaking or resting. This embrace releases the groin and hips, draws circulation through the sex organs and glands, eases the low back and promotes perfect union.

Try rocking forward and back and side to side. Explore and see what is there for you.

Repeat for the other partner.

RESTING POSE
Your resting posture is the most important of all you have done.

It is here in stillness that you actually receive the benefits of every twist and turn, posture and hold, breath and sigh.

As you relax, all of the life force opened through each posture sings through the body and the mind, touching every cell with the kiss of vitality.

As you rest together you continue to move into sync.

Your peace adds to your partner's peace, energy to energy, joy to joy, and love to love until you are both complete.

Both of you whole, both of you healthy, both of you perfect in this

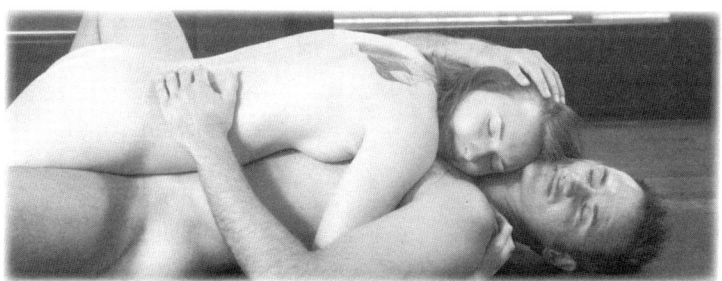

Chapter 8: The Chakras
Experienced through Meditation, Yoga
Postures and Intimate Chakra Massage

To completely comprehend the chakras would be to unravel the mysteries of the Universe through the act of self knowing.

The chakra system is a vast topic deserving more than our light touch. The exercises in this chapter can be viewed as a simple entry to something rich and sometimes mysterious. Practice the exercises with an open mind and heart. Your own experience will be your best teacher.

The word chakra means "wheel of light." They are not made of matter but instead represent a confluence of life force energies. When these energies combine, they act as a portal between the overlapping dimensions of mind and body, matter and spirit.

As a rudimentary example, imagine this:

You are standing in front of a large window inside the heart of your home. From where you stand you are able to extend a part of your awareness into all you see within your field of vision and in some way sense what lies beyond it. The window also allows light to fill your home from sources of energy as far away as the Sun, the Moon, and starry galaxies beyond.

The chakras act much like a window by allowing a crossover between the unseen dimensions of our extended energy field to merge with the flesh and bone reality of our innermost core.

This is the connective tissue that carries the consciousness of the soul through to its denser expression as manifested by the body.

The seven major chakras each have a physical reference point along the length of the spine which acts as a conduit for this non-physical part of our anatomy.

They each vibrate at the subtle frequencies of sound and light, and it is the presence of the chakras that creates an open dialogue between mind, body and soul, the domain of one bearing a direct influence upon the others.

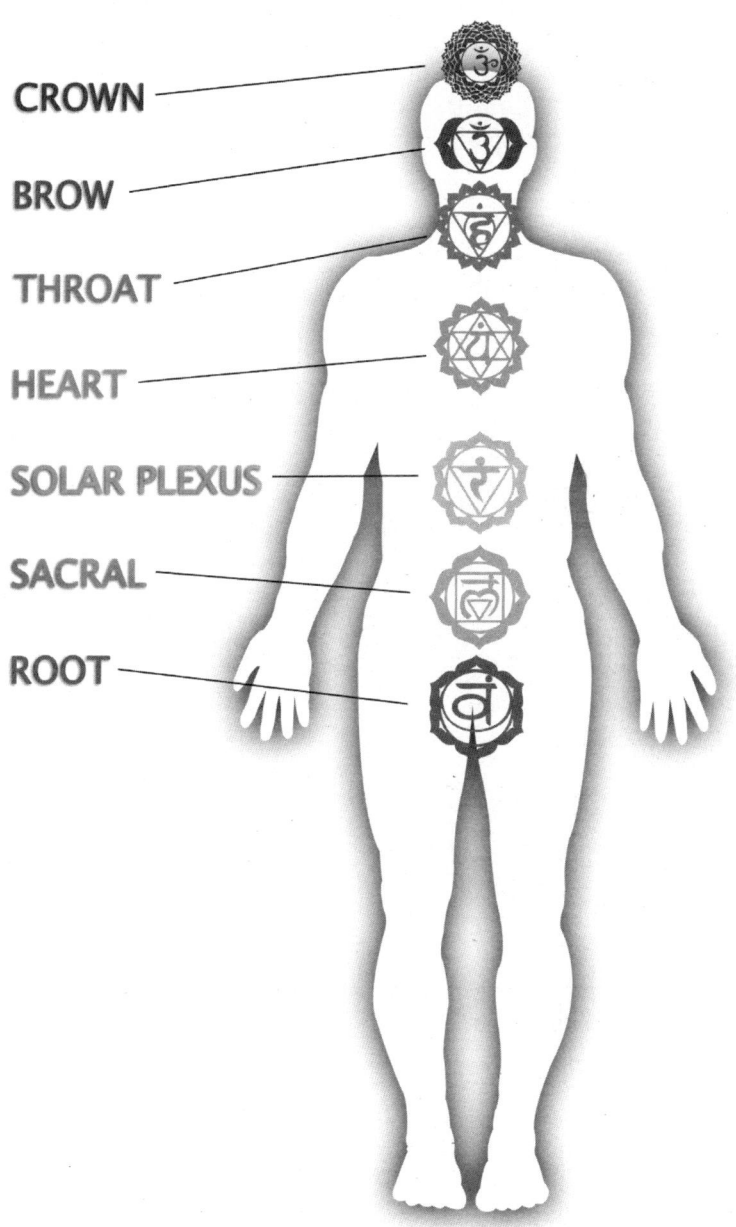

Seen by those with the gift of clairvoyance as wheels of pulsing light, the chakras are felt most clearly through the effects of their balance or imbalance as experienced through our relationship to life, the appearance of our bodies and the ever changing landscape of our thoughts and emotions.

We can hear them speak through bodily sensations, glimpses of intuition, insight and increased awareness.

We can touch them with meditation and with visualizations... ...with will, wish and imagination...

...with the current of sound as intoned with your voice, and with the physical postures of yoga.

Archetypally, the chakras reflect the natural world around us by holding at heart the essence of the elements: Earth, Water, Fire, Air, Sound, Light, and Space.

Each of us is a balance of strengths and weaknesses that together make a whole and interesting individual. As we become familiar with the chakras we can begin to see which have the strongest influences in how we approach the relationships in our lives and how our relationship to survival, sexuality, power, love, etc. create the life we live and the people who are the major players in it.

How will this heat up your sex life?

Speaking to their physiological ties, the seven major chakras have a direct correspondence to glands in the endocrine system, which is vital to our sexual health.

Root - Sex Glands

Sacral - Adrenals

Solar Plexus - Pancreas

Heart - Thymus

Throat - Thyroid

Brow - Pituitary

Crown - Pineal

These glands produce powerful hormones which regulate your metabolism, vitality, libido, and emotional equilibrium. When this system is out of balance your quality of life can suffer tremendously. The good news - with a little understanding your yoga practice can become an act of self rejuvenation. As you learn to feel or visualize the energy fields around each chakra center your endocrine system is washed with subtle energy called prana or life force.

The addition of yoga postures aimed at detoxifying your organs and juicing up your glands will have lasting results far more satisfying than a pricey trip to the day spa or another refill for that Viagra prescription. As you know, great sex has its roots in a healthy body - the sizzle of raw physical sensuality is a potent aphrodisiac. The fact that your endocrine system is inextricably entwined to the balance of your mood and emotions points out another intriguing factor tying the function of the chakras to the sexy integration of body mind and soul.

On a more subtle level:
Great sex is also about freely exchanging energy. We become a portal to each other, feeling the other through our own skin, feeling ourselves in the response of our partner, picking up information through subtle and not so subtle cues. The delicious experience of perfect oneness has everything to do with the open flow of energy through and between the chakras - yours and your partner's in harmonious spin.

As an opening example let's consider the Heart chakra. It is here that the physical act of sex meets the non-physical domain of love. A clear heart center is what makes sex and orgasm more than athletics with a short lived bang of pleasure. Both the feeling of your heart overflowing with emotion, and the melting sensation of dissolving boundaries, bear the signature of a healthy heart center.

When the powerful desire to merge takes hold, it is this chakra that allows wish fulfillment. Both in physical form, as our bodies move into sexual embrace, and multi-dimensional, as the flow of positive energies generated in the first three chakras moves through the transformative chamber of the heart to expand as the rarified light of love, freedom, and yes, ecstasy.

A focus on the chakras encourages examining the patterns of thought and behaviors that live there. By learning to clear and balance the chakras, your sexual experiences will become richer as you become more sensitive to the energetic charge and the attitudes that are contained by each.

A good example lies in the heart of our ability or inability to enjoy sex without inhibition. When you begin to heal the second chakra, your thoughts and feelings about sex will likely rise to the surface. If you find lurking shadows of shame, guilt or other trauma, the second chakra holds the keys to freeing yourself from the past.

As you release old attitudes about love and relationships that no longer serve you, the way becomes open to deeper emotional connection and sexual freedom. Your couple's yoga practice supports heightened sensitivity to one another, better communication, and an increase in trust and intimacy as you continue to grow in love and joy.

Working with the chakras

The practices herein are organized as a sequence of experiences that begin with the subtle elements of breath, life force, and visualization - gradually following the path of gravitational pull towards finding physical manifestation through the joys of shared postures, touch, and sensual pleasure.

A yoga practice at heart holds the intention of awakening the potential - human and divine - sleeping within. The chakras hold the seeds of this awakening.

In making a beginning let us start here...

The Chakras with correspondences and points of contact
Become familiar with each chakra before continuing on. Give voice to each name, sound each syllable, and touch each colorful location with both the fingers of your hand and the fingers of your focus.

Visualize the physical expression of each chakra as stepping stones marking an ascendant path from your perineum to the crown of your head.

Opening Your Luminous Core Meditation

This first exercise establishes an awareness of the chakras and the currents of innate energy that flow through and around the central core of your being.

-Sit comfortably alone or in any comfortable position with your partner.

-Drop into a steady natural breath. By following the breath as it comes and goes, one can tap into the feeling of upward current with the inhalation and downward current with the breath exhaled.

-Stay inside this simple focus until the breath feels smooth and deep. Allow a feeling of effortlessness to bring ease to your body and mind as the breath travels up and down, in and out.

-Imagine a luminous channel or pathway that runs from the area of your perineum directly through to the top of your head.

-Imagine seeing light filling your body from the root of the perineum to the opening at the crown of your head. As you exhale, imagine the light and energy returning to the earth, carried on the sound of your sigh.

Stay inside this simple focus until the energy you are observing feels unbroken - its journey experienced as a steady stream of light and sensation. As this becomes clearly felt or even seen with your inner sight - insight - you will have opened your luminous core.

This channel of energy guides the powerhouse of our raw physical energy upward toward the refining process of the upper chakras. It also brings the insight and spirit of the upper chakras to earth, where they manifest through our physical body in all we do. This is also the trail that our orgasmic energies follow as they reach toward the taste of bliss.

The yogic term for this channel is the Shushumna.

The Shushumna is the energetic stem that holds the petal blooms of the chakras. As each chakra absorbs cosmic vibrations, the Shushumna distributes them as needed throughout the body/mind.

As you do the exercise you may become aware of light and vibration felt as warm tingling along the spine.

Where your focus goes is where the life force follows. As you imagine drawing your breath up the center of the Shushumna with the inhalation, you are indeed flooding this pathway with intelligence and energy. As you drop into your breathing, let the breath itself open this sacred pathway.

Later as you follow the exercise, breathing into each chakra flower, you are allowing your gentle focus to clear the static from the subtle circuitry of the chakra and its field of influence. Later, as you learn to send your awareness through the chakras to merge with your partner, you will notice that there is a tangible shift toward a deeper sense of connectedness.

With practice you may begin to notice where you feel restricted or less open and where you can expand freely. When a chakra is restricted, its expression in our life is thrown out of balance. Tuning your senses to the quality of each chakra is the first step toward recognizing and healing imbalance.

The light of your awareness and the prana inside of each breath is nourishing in ways that food and rest are not. In relationship to our sexual nature, the rising energy that flows through our luminous stem must pierce each of the chakras as it ascends the spinal cord. In this way it can reach the brain's central nervous system and endocrine center - the hypothalamus and pituitary gland - which ignite the spark of hormonal magic that supports our sexual health and blesses our lives with longevity and joy.

Chakra Mala Meditation
Use what you have learned in the last meditation to enter this one together.

Many meditation practices are done in rounds. A round is made up of a series of focuses, breaths, mantras, or counts.

Traditionally, a necklace of beads is used to count off each breath, one bead passed through your fingers with the utterance of each seed syllable. This necklace is called a Mala.

In this visualization we will imagine the chakras as beautiful gemstones making a mala. Holding each one with the fingers of your focus, travel from the root chakra to the crown.

Complete the cycle by continuing back from the crown to the root chakra, thus completing one round of focused meditation.

Touching the Chakras - Visualization

EXERCISE KEY ◙ ○ •
◙ **means working in unison**
○ **means SHE moves**
• **means HE moves**

◙ Sit back-to-back with your partner.
◙ Tune into the rhythm of your breathing - fall into harmony.
◙ Press the length of your spines together.
◙ Notice the pulse of awareness quickening inside the spine.
◙ Let your breath slowly open your luminous core.
◙ Sit as one, following the feeling and sound of each cycle of breath.
◙ Notice as the rivers of your life force flow together, making one strong current between you.

Hold this pattern of breath and focus until the sense of connection is strong. Tell your partner what you are feeling. When you are in agreement, shift the breath pattern as follows:

◙ Inhale as if through the front of your body – filling completely.
◙ Exhale through your back - sending yourself through your partner.
◙ Use this basic breath to draw your senses powerfully inside.
◙ Feel the intelligence communicating through your cells as your life force moves beyond physical boundaries to the experience of union.

◉ Hold this pattern of breath and focus until you are completely engaged with the life force of breath and sensation. Let thought drop away.

Begin the Chakra Mala Meditation
◉ Drop your awareness to the floor of your body - finding the pulse of your Root chakra.
◉ With the fingers of your focus, touch the garnet bead of the Muladhara/Root chakra.
◉ Inhale as if through the crown of your head - connecting with the Root chakra at the floor of your body - charging this center with garnet red glow.
◉ Exhale - expanding through yourself to your partner - combining your energies and light as one... a big red blaze of Root chakra joy!
◉ Pause here for several full cycles of breath - sharing the glow - the radiance of this gemstone coming clearly into view, its color softly lighting the space between your brows.

Progress upward through the chakras one at a time, continuing on in the same breathing rhythm, holding each focus for several full cycles of breath. Drop your awareness to the physical location, finding its pulse with the fingers of your focus.

◉ Touch the carnelian bead of the Swadhisthana/Sacral chakra - charge it with red orange glow.

◉ Pick up the topaz bead of the Manipurna/Solar Plexus chakra - charge it with rich yellow glow.

◉ Touch the emerald bead of the Anahata/Heart chakra - charge it with verdant green glow.

◉ Touch the turquoise bead of the Vishuddha/Throat chakra - charge it with sky blue glow.

◉ Move to the star sapphire bead of the Ajna/Brow chakra - charge it with indigo glow.

◉ Touch the diamond bead of the Sahasrara/Crown chakra - charge it with unearthly light.

Hold here for seven cycles of breath. Absorb the cosmic energies from all around you, reaching through the light of this chakra to tap into its higher source. Repeat this mala, descending from top to bottom. Hold at the bottom for seven cycles of breath, grounding the awakened prana at the root of your being.

Touching the Chakras - Sound
You can add the vibration of sound to this exercise using the traditional bij mantras or vowel sounds which occur in our mother tongue. They are listed in our previous reference chart. The yogis use sound/mantra to further direct the focus of the mind.

Chanting a mantra may make it easier for you to feel a sense of connection with the focus of your meditation. As sound travels from the resonant caverns of your body to enter the atmosphere, it makes its presence known through the life force resident inside the breath, and the specific vibration it carries. The vehicle of the mantra/sound provides a strong focus for the mind.

Bij mantras and seed syllables resonate at the same frequency as the vibrational body of each chakra. Tones carried upon the breath, or sustained as soundless sound within the mind, create a resonant harmony that brings healing balance. Consider one round of this meditation to be made of twenty-one counts, contacting each chakra three times before lifting your focus to the next.

- Use the inhaled breath to draw your awareness within, anchoring your focus.

- Use the exhaled breath to voice your mantra/vowel, spinning the breath out as a long gossamer thread, a delicate circuitry of sound, vibration and light moving you to yet another layer of deep connection and balance.

- To finish, chant the sound of AUM three times, sealing yourselves to the sound of universal harmony.

- Rest in silence, listening for the echo of its effect.

Over time the chakras will unfold like a flower in slow bloom to reveal its many petals. Each of us is unique in our ability to sense, feel, and see into the subtle energy systems of the body. Much of this information speaks to us from in between the layers of the conscious and subconscious mind.

In touching a chakra, one person may actually see a color behind their shuttered lids, while another will only imagine the color but feel warmth or gentle pressure around the physical contact of the chakra held in focus.

One person will have flashes of insight - an ultra knowing or epiphany - that resolves a long held pattern, while another will experience the emotions that are governed therein.

It is best to approach with a quiet mind, emptied of expectation, open to what "is." As the chakras uncoil, spiritual energies are freed to flow through every system of your body. Your emotions now soar toward their highest aspects and your mind is blessed with greater light - entrained by the transcendent aspiration of your soul.

Touching the Chakras - The Postures
We now shift our focus to the temple of the body, bringing all the awareness gained into our house.

In this phase, what was thought and spirit becomes manifest through our touch, postures, and actions. Our sense of unity is now expressed in the solid reality of our connection. Each posture is an archetype, reflecting our relationship to universal themes.

Imagine your postures as sacred symbols – Yantras – which form a bridge between the worlds, evoking the soul of each chakra as deity, stretching from inside your every cell to reach into the infinite wisdom of the universe.

"Nobody can go to heaven unless the foundation is firm." B. K. S. Iyengar

ROOT CHAKRA - MULADHARA

The qualities of this chakra are stability, stillness, peace and an ability to thrive that comes from very deep roots.

It is here that we find our connection to the physical world and from here that we draw our ability to survive, have self-confidence, and know that we have the right to *BE*.

The following posture expresses these qualities by making a firm foundation of your bodies joined.

DOUBLE CHAIR POSE

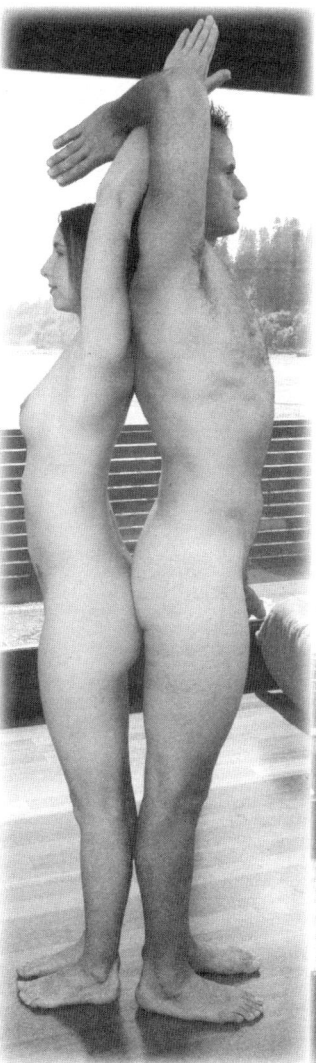

◙ From standing, extend your Namaste one to another.

◙ Turn back-to-back, connecting firmly from shoulders to hips.

◙ Link arms and bend your knees, bringing your thighs to a parallel alignment to the floor.

◙ Follow the flow or gravity, extending the length of the exhaled breath.

◙ Absorb the stability in your pose as you descend to seated.

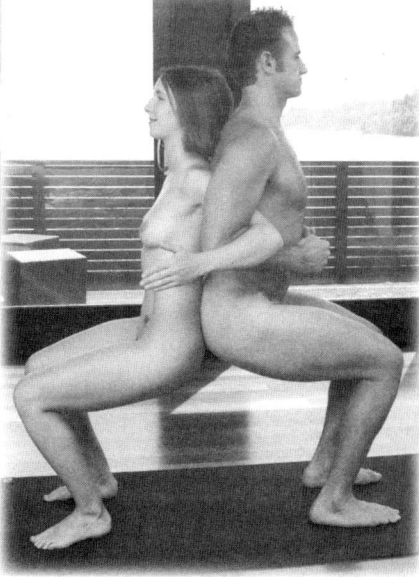

- Contact the earth with your sit bones, perineum, and planted feet.

- Meet your partner with solid contact, your backs like unshakeable bedrock.

- Rest your foundation on the foundation of the earth.

- Be there.

Affirmation - "We are"

Bij mantra - Circulate the vibration of "Lam" as sound or sustained inside the mind

Visualize - Red ember glow

Experience - Stability/peace

SACRAL CHAKRA – SWADHISTHANA

It is here we come in contact with our innate need for community, for each other. This chakra governs emotions, creativity and the expression of our sexuality, and opens to the great gift of giving and receiving pleasure, nurture and life. Pleasure frees the body from tension and invites relaxation.

As we enter relaxation together, we open through the body to the subtle energies pulsing from this chakra as warm widening waves.

The following posture makes a deep basin for the sea of life in the depths of the sacrum. Your spine will act as a long wave of connection, potent with pleasure and deep with peace.

DOUBLE GODDESS POSE
- Turn face to face. Separate your legs side to side and scoot forward.
- Bend your knees to plant the soles of your feet to either side of your partner's waist.
- Lie back on the floor.
- Allow your heavy knees to open out to the sides.

◉ Rest the pleasant weight of your legs inside your partner's inner thighs, bringing release to her hips and sacrum.
◉ Let the warm cradle of your thighs give him permission to relax completely into your support.

◉ Hold here, or complete the pose by bringing the soles of your feet together to rest on your partner's abdomen.

◉ Together, begin to follow the impulse of each breath to create a long wave of slow pleasure.

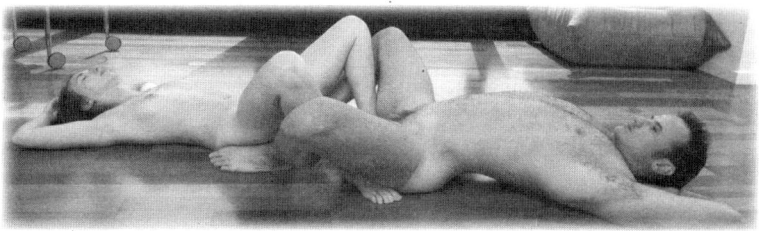

◉ Inhale, rocking your tailbone toward the floor - low back lifting from the floor.
◉ Imagine pouring into the warm sea of life force inside the circle of your entwined thighs.
◉ Exhale, rocking your tailbone upward - low back pressing the floor below.
◉ Imagine the warm sea of life force pouring into you.
◉ Hold this rhythm, allowing your spines to generate heat, finding the pulse inside of each breath.

To deepen your connection...
○ Inhales, rocking her tailbone forward, while...
● Exhales, pressing his low back to the floor.
◉ Share the inverted breath as your rhythm, pouring into each other in turn.

Your breath and movement in opposition make a long fluid infinite loop of your energy and produce a strong sensation of pleasure. Pleasure opens your whole system to a vital state of flow, as we relax and surrender to its touch.

Affirmation - "We create"

Visualize - Orange fluid waves

Bij mantra - Circulate the sound or soundless vibration "Vwam"

Experience - Pleasure/connection

SUPINE STRADDLE POSE
This continues to energize the Swadhisthana chakra. The mutual support here is quite freeing and relaxing to the groin and sexual organs.

- From Double Goddess pose, simply straighten your legs.
- Rest your feet together, one partner outside, the other inside.
- Allow your legs to open out to the sides. The inside partner rests completely into the support of the outside partner.

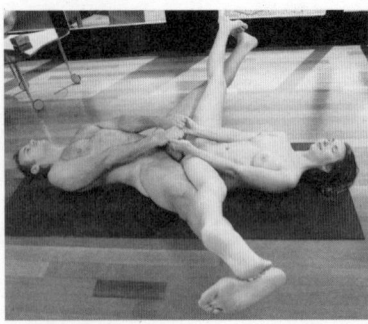
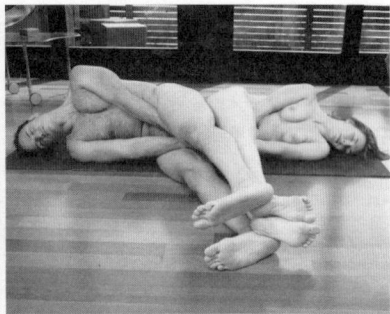

Hold here for several cycles of breath.

Add rocking side to side for a playful variation. This deeply cleanses tension from the sacrum and groin areas while encouraging blood flow to the sex centers of your bodies.

SOLAR PLEXUS CHAKRA - MANIPURNA

Here we resonate to the qualities of will and forward motion, overcoming inertia to find power in the assertion of selves. This center takes warmth and fans it to a fire, burning off dross to encourage clarity of focus and a strength
of direction.

Centered behind your navel, this area holds the strength of your character and an abundance of vitality. In this posture we make a push in one direction, joining our strengths with joyful determination.

DOUBLE BRIDGE POSE
◙ From Supine Straddle Pose, both partners bend their legs and plant their feet firmly to the floor, a hip width apart.
• One partner places his feet on top of the other's bent knees.

◙ Together - Inhale, pressing down through the length of your arms and the palms of your hands to find the power to lift, thighs, hips, belly and chest toward the sun.
◙ Exhale, relaxing your low back to the floor.

◙ Repeat three times. Follow your breath into the heat of your will, drinking in the vitality available to strengthen your shared foundation.

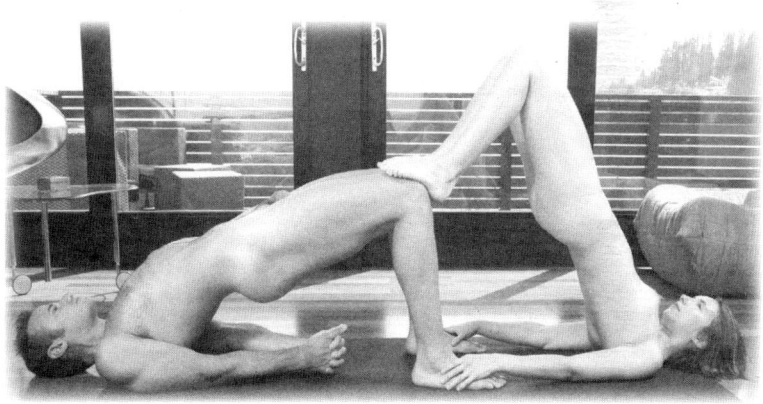

Trade positions with your partner and repeat three times.

Affirmation - "We can"

Visualize - Golden glowing rays

Bij mantra - Circulate the sound or soundless vibration "Ram"

Experience - Heat/vitality

This posture also stimulates the upper chakra centers as energies and circulation flow in an upward rising direction.

Modification:
Make a gentle push upward, lifting your hips slightly off the floor. This takes less energy and removes any strain from the arms, shoulders, or wrists.

HEART CHAKRA - ANAHATA

Here we find the home of both passionate and spiritual love, joyful expression, and the gift of compassion. This chakra governs the lungs, heart, arms and hands. Breath and spirit merge bringing the sensation of expanding joy. Our arms embrace all of humanity and our hands open with selfless giving.

In this posture we free the chest and unburden the heart, leaving us light enough to enter the magnetism of the upper chakras.

CHILD'S POSE WITH SUPINE CAMEL POSE
- From Double Bridge Pose, return to sitting face to face.
- From seated, move to Child's Pose. Make yourself comfortable. Settle in, allowing your forehead to rest on the floor and your hips to relax toward your heels.

- Move to kneeling behind your partner's hips, turning your back to him. Your feet will be to the outside of his hips. Use your hands to slowly lower your back onto the support of his. The back of your heart should center at the mid to low end of his scapula. Your head will nest at his shoulders. Let go into his support. Breathe deeply, letting the breath continue to open your heart. Move your arms anywhere they feel comfortable. You can maximize the heart aspects of this posture by letting your arms open out to the sides in pure surrender like wings, or reach up and overhead to create a stronger back bend.

- Continue to lift your heart and release with each breath, opening like a rose in full bloom, your hands sliding slowly down the length of your partner's arms until finding the grasp of his waiting hands.

- Hold for several cycles of breath before reversing, exchanging roles and repeating for the other partner.

Affirmation - "We love"

Visualize - Green or rose light opening as a many-petaled bloom

Bij Mantra - Circulate the sound or soundless vibration "Yam"

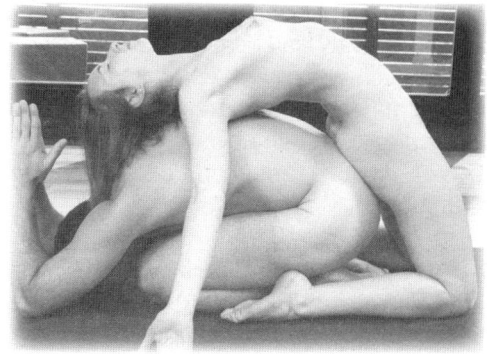

Experience - Freedom/full acceptance

Modification:
If the back bend in this posture is too strong, move your knees and hips further away from the direction of your partner's head before you begin to lay back.

THROAT CHAKRA - VISHUDDHA

In this center, will takes on the form of self-expression, giving voice to your thoughts with clear communication. Our ability to communicate brings us out of isolation, our consciousness moving towards unity through shared dreams. This chakra assimilates and transmits knowledge, this knowledge taking on creative dimensions as valuable ideas are brought to manifestation by speaking them, and following with actions of the same quality and direction. Here we learn that a word has power - to build up or tear down, yourself or your world. "I love" creates and "I hate" destroys.

The word "Vishuddha" means purification. The energies freed in the lower chakras rise to be purified by fire. Transformation occurs as the matter-generated flames produce something finer - the light of your growing consciousness. As our consciousness elevates, we naturally shift away from the coarse, heavy vibrations of hatred and anger. We become skilled at directing our thoughts and speech in positive ways - transforming both self and society.

This posture sends nourishment and life force to the area of the throat, pituitary and heart. We assist each other into the posture using touch, sensitivity, and full presence as communication skills. When the posture is released, we find freedom from tension, clarity of mind, and more depth of heart, making our voice deep with its own unique resonance. Say "Haahhhmmmm" and hear the difference.

PLOW POSE - ARDHA HALASANA

- Lay down side by side, shoulder to shoulder, with your feet extending in opposite directions.

- Bend both knees and draw them to your chest.

- Place your palms firmly to the Earth at either side of your hips. Press down into your hands as you slowly straighten your legs. Your hips will lift from the floor as you continue to reach back through your toes in the direction of your head.

- Roll backward into Plow Pose as your toes find the floor.

- Lift your hands to your low back for support as your hips align with one another. Draw your chin toward your chest and your chest toward your chin.

- Move your focus deeply inside the experience of the breath circulating throughout the posture. Feel the interior spaces of your body expand with each breath. Note the pulse at the base of your throat. Imagine replenishing this center with the light of your focus and the gift of the posture.

- Try chanting the sound of OM together. This further stimulates and clears the throat center and adds another dimension of connection between the two of you as your voices join as one voice, one vibration and one unified field of energy.

Rest here for seven cycles of breath before rolling down one vertebra at a time.

Affirmation - "We speak"

Color - Clear Blue Beam

Bij Mantra - Circulate the sound or soundless vibration "Ham"

Experience - Resonance/clarity

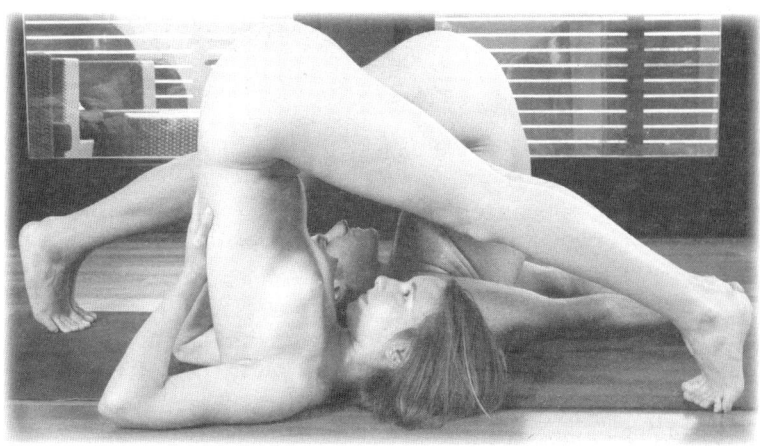

Modification:
To protect a vulnerable neck or a less flexible spine:

Roll back only far enough to place your hands under your hips for support. Keep both knees softly bent.

Relax the weight of your legs rather than extending them back.

BROW CHAKRA - AJNA and CROWN CHAKRA - SAHASRARA

In these two chakras we find the inner eye opening to what was previously unseen, as we lift our gaze to the inner life of the soul. The realm of intuition, inspiration, dreams, visions, and rational thought, it is here we link mind, body and spirit with the super consciousness of the universal mind. We develop the gift of sight, looking both outward and inward. Insight and perception are now the guiding lanterns with which we chart our course.

In this Double Savasana we can absorb or follow the flow of rising consciousness from root to crown, where in resting we receive new vision. As you rest, allow the flow of awareness to move gently through the two upper chakras. Imagine lifting your inner gaze or insight upward, the way you would if you were to lift your physical eyes upward to gaze at the fullest moon casting its light through the night sky.

DOUBLE SAVASANA

- From facing one another, lie down with your legs extended towards your partner in an open V shape.
- Scoot close enough to allow your feet to easily make contact with your partner's hands.
- Gently rest your feet in the upturned palms of your partner, making a closed circuitry of connection for the life force and expansion you have released.
- Observe and absorb this energy by noticing the sensations in your body - feelings of openness and space, freeing the body and the mind.
- Imagine floating together, drifting on each breath, as if supported by an infinite sea of contentment - whole, perfect and at peace.
- Rest until you feel a sense of being complete.

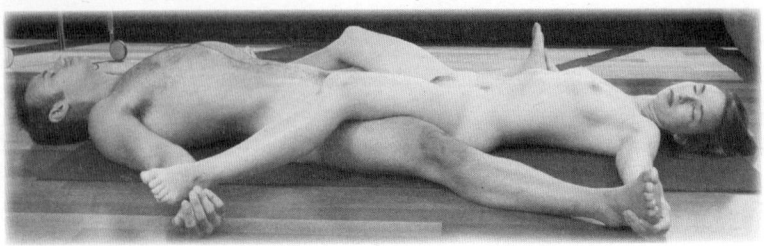

For the Ajna or Brow center:
Affirmation - "We see"

Color - Indigo expanse

Bij mantra - Circulate the sound or the soundless vibration "Sham". "Om" also works here.

Experience - Inner sight/sensation = experience of merging dimensions

For the Sahasara or Crown center:

Affirmation - "We expand"

Colors - Violet to White

Bij Mantra - Circulate the sound or soundless vibration "Om"

Experience - Expanding consciousness/universal connection/bliss

CHAKRA MASSAGE
Taking the experience deeper still

Follow the upward drift of your partner's energy with sensitive touch and practiced awareness.

To begin, the partner taking the active - or serving - roll sits on the floor, legs stretched out side by side. The receiving partner turns to lie down with back resting across thighs, head to the right and feet to the left, pillow placed under the head for comfort.

This experience can take anywhere from 15 minutes to an hour, depending on your mood and ability to hold focus for a longer period of time. Be sure you are comfortable, adjusting the room temperature to be comfortable in the nude. Have water or tea nearby so when thirsty you can drink without losing connectionor focus with your partner. The active partner may also enjoy a pillow beneath his sit bones for additional support.

Establishing clear connection:

- The active partner should take a moment to fall into sync with himself, moving inside to his own sense of center one focused breath at a time.
- From where you are - Repeat the Luminous Core Meditation for a few minutes until a strong connection is felt to your own life force and energy.

Contacting the Root Chakra
- Lean slightly forward, placing your hand in the area of the root chakra between the perineum and the genitals. Place your other hand gently on the heart center.

- Keeping the hand over the heart still, pulse your other hand

with the rhythm of
the breath, pressing
gently upward with
the inhaled breath
and releasing with the
exhaled sigh. Hold
here for a minimum of
seven cycles of breath,
gradually building up
to five minutes. Use
this as your rhythm
throughout the exercise.

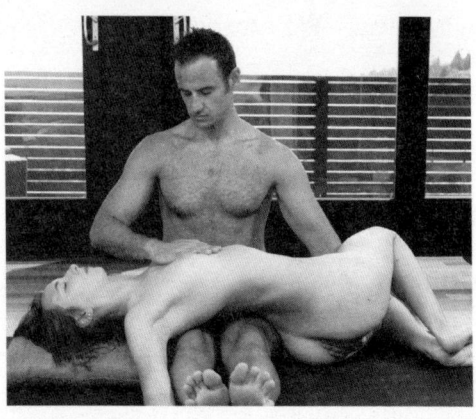

○ Receiving partner - You can intensify your connection to the root chakra and its pulse. Contract the muscles of the perineum and "lift" the pelvic floor with the ascendant inhaled breath, and relax with the exhaled breath.

You may wish to continue this pulse throughout the exercise to consciously direct the flow of your prana upward.

Contacting the Sacral Chakra
• Giving partner - Move your hand to rest across the genitals - over the mound of the pubic bone, or lightly across his genitals.

• Follow the rhythm of your breathing as you gently rock your hand side to side. Move from your own sense of center, your whole body participating in this touch.

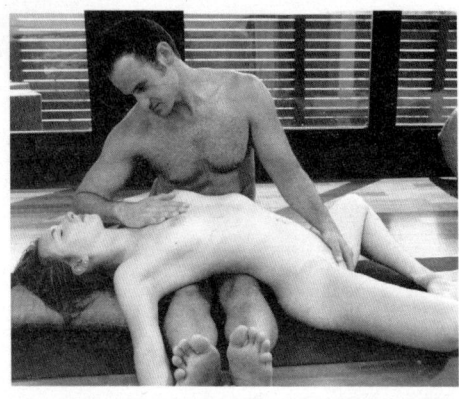

• Hold here for seven cycles of breath.

Contacting the Solar Plexus Chakra
• Move your hand to your partner's solar plexus, spanning the gap

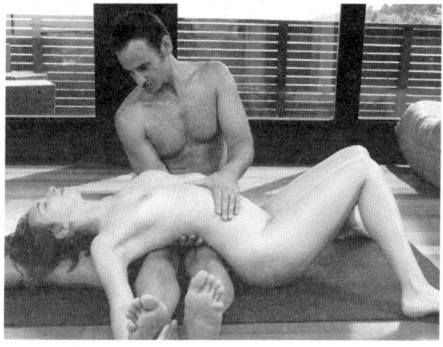

between the navel and the heart.

- Moving from your own center, make slow circles seven times, rolling around the full surface of your palm.

- Repeat in the opposite direction.

This releases core tension and opens the emotions to a deep even flow in the direction of the heart.

Contacting the Heart Chakra
- Move both hands to rest on the heart center.

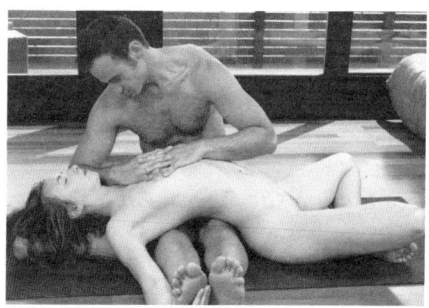

- Leave your hands here until your feel a pure sense of connection.

- Be a conduit for the profound gift of unconditional love.

Contacting the Throat Chakra
- Brush your fingers to your partner's throat center. One hand can return to the heart.

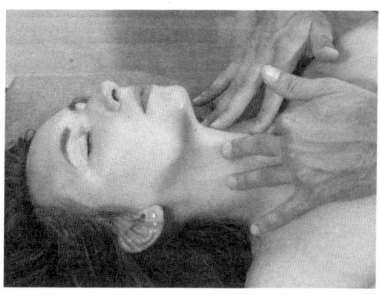

- Let this change of position indicate a
major shift of awareness - the integration of the lower chakras with the consciousness reaching in from the higher chakras.

- Rest here for seven cycles of breath, both partners humming softly with each exhaled breath, the resonance speaking to the mind of your fingertips.

Contacting the Third Eye Chakra
- Rub your palms together vigorously, lighting a small fire between them.

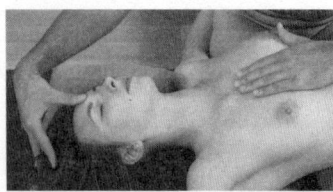

- Shake all the excess energy from your hands, scattering sparks to all four corners.

- Lift your hands and rest them both over your partner's eyes. This anchors the sight to the inner world, all cares vanishing in the knowing of peace.

- Hold here for seven cycles of breath.

- Gradually slide one hand back down to her heart while gently moving your thumb to rest at the point between her eyebrows, stimulating the third eye directly.

Contacting the Crown Chakra
Here we open to the bliss nature of the soul as available to our bodies through the governing aspect of enlightened thought. It is to this point that all of our energies aspire.

It is here that we reach to find the next rung of a ladder now invisible, as we have moved into the realm of the soul and its source.

The posture here reflects openness and invites absorption, the whole body relaxed and thrumming with life, the sound of "Om" emanating from every pore.

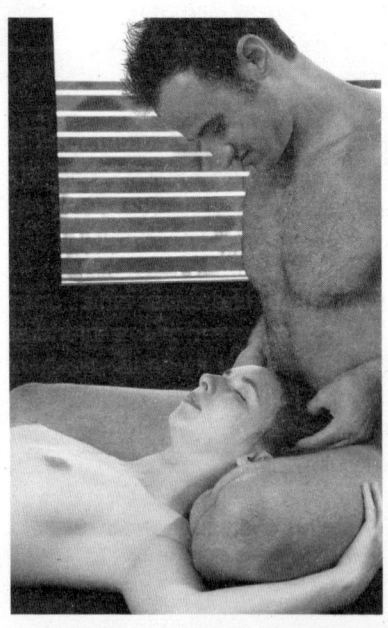

- Active partner - slowly shift your position to seated at her head.

- Sit comfortably with your legs crossed, or extend your legs down either side of her body, adding a sense of sweet nurturing containment to this open posture of mind and heart.

- Hold your fingertips just beneath the occipital ridge at the base of the cranium. You will feel two soft points around the area where the second or middle fingers are curled beneath the bony ridge of the cranium.
- Let the weight of her head settle into your fingertips.
- Imagine that as you inhale you are drawing her energies upward beyond the crown.
- As you exhale, send a wave of unconditional love from your heart through your hands, washing every cell with violet glow.

- Take time to fall into your breathing, moving into harmony within yourself and with your partner.
- Enjoy the free flow of life force stretching from pole to pole, from head to toes, from one to the other.
- Ride this pulse to touch every cell of your being - falling into harmony with all that is.

- Relax. Fix your gaze between your brows or lift them to observe the clear center of the moon
illuminating the sky of your mind.

- Let your gaze lift you higher, becoming absorbed by the light inside your opening crown.

Affirmation - "We know"

Color - Violet white

Bij mantra - Circulate the sound or soundless vibration "Om" or the vowel sound "nnnggg"

Experience - Deepest peace/transcendent being

Chapter 9: Life in Balance
Postures, Breathing, Massage and Sexual Practices for Total Well-Being

I've mentioned "balancing the chakras" a number of times. What is balance?

A balanced chakra functions like a top in perfect spin. It hums with energy and holds its position steady within its gravitational field. Imagine seven spinning tops humming with positive vibration, generating a field of light and sound around them. The rainbow of their individual colors overlap as energy is effectively transmitted from one to the next, creating a resonant chord - a subtle OM - connecting each to the celestial song of the Universe. This is balance.

Now picture one top losing its energy. Struggling to spin it wobbles wildly, making lose sloppy circles.

Another spins far too fast, skipping out of bounds and dispersing heat. As the steady stream of light and vibration becomes erratic, the other spinning spheres are pulled out of alignment.

When one chakra is out of balance the whole system compensates by becoming somewhat excessive or deficient as a new pulse emerges - making an uneasy balance from discordant notes.

Now apply the image of a top moving out of spin to your root chakra. A wobbling top here would radically shift your feelings of rootedness, security and physical energy. Imagine another top in rapid spin in the upper chakra centers. This would have a profound effect on your thoughts, clarity of mind and ability to focus.

When the mind is in overdrive it usually fails to connect with positive or physical action. Instead we get caught in fruitless daydreaming or procrastination, or become irritable and anxious.

Chakra imbalances are most easily understood as they manifest in our thoughts, emotions and behavior. An open or restricted chakra can have a heavy impact on your relationships with others, and more importantly with yourself.

The nature and influence of the chakras is a vast area of study. In an effort to simplify, making balance easier to grasp and imbalance just a momentary wobble in time, let's go back to the five basic elements.

Five Element Theory

The same five elements that make up the Universe also govern our human physiology. If you are paying attention, the innate qualities of earth, water, fire, air, and space are easily relatable to the basic makeup of our mind/body constitution.

Earth. Body, muscles, bone, the gift of abundance, vitality, and a lust for life.

Water. Sex organs, all watery substances in the body, circulation, the gift of creativity, sexuality, movement and change.

Fire. Adrenal glands, pancreas "hot organs" (such liver, gall bladder, digestion) the gift of a passionate personality, power, and personal will.

Air. Thyroid and thymus glands; the breath itself, the gift of speech, creative communication, open-heartedness, the spaciousness of joy, and love.

Space. Governs Pituitary, Pineal, and Hypothalamus glands; consciousness, a bright mind, the ability to think, dream, and imagine.

They also bear direct correspondence to the Chakras:

Earth - Root Chakra
Water - Sacral Chakra
Fire - Solar Plexus Chakra
Air - Heart and Throat Chakras
Space - Third Eye to Crown Chakras

Every element is a vital powerhouse that supports our human experience, but - our theory in a nutshell - too much of any good thing can wreak havoc in your life if left unchecked. The good news is that once you are able to recognize imbalance at its root, you have the ability to bring yourself back to a place of inner peace and relative sanity with your yoga practice.

The following postures are grouped according to the corresponding element they most directly affect. In seeking balance, a basic guideline to follow is this: When there is a deficiency or excess of an element, it is treated with a dose of its opposite or complementary element. For example, if you are feeling anxious, irritable and spacey, you may be experiencing excessive Air and Space. Try postures for the Earth and/or Water elements to both ground and soothe yourself.

Earth Element Postures:
Seated Forward Bend
Child's Pose
Knees to Chest Pose
Bridge Pose

Instructions for the postures above are in Chapter 6 and Chapter 7. They all emphasize a grounded connection to the Earth.

Forward Bends like Child's Pose and Seated Forward Bend draw the awareness within while making relaxation almost effortless. Bridge Pose places your feet firmly on the earth for stability, while Knees to Chest Pose offers perfect support to a place that often craves it - your back.

Water Element Postures:
Sacral Rocking
Knees to Chest Pose
Pigeon Pose
Cat Stretches

Water postures invite a sense of flow. They also target the hips and groin areas associated with our sexual core.

Fire Element Postures:
Energizing Breath
Upward Facing Dog
Downward Facing Dog

Warrior One
Seated Breath of Fire

Fire postures develop strength and warm the body.

Air Element Postures:
Camel Pose
Downward Facing Dog
Triangle Pose
Warrior Two

Air postures open the chest, heart and lungs. All of these poses address freedom and openness in different ways. Feel it to understand.

Space Element Postures:
Seated Meditation
Tree Pose
Eagle Pose
Triangle

Space opens up from a place of pure focus. These postures all require your complete presence to the present moment and that alone.

Be here and now - not anywhere else.

As you choose elements to work with, the corresponding chakras will also benefit.

Another interesting fact about the elements is that when they are combined they make up 3 distinct personality types. These personality types are called Doshas.

When Earth and Water are paired they make a Kapha type.

When Water and Fire are combined they create a Pitta personality.

When Space and Air are coupled we have a Vata point of view.

We all inherit a unique mix of these three mind/body principles which govern our dominant mental and physical characteristics.

In getting to know your elemental personality type you can more easily assess what is out of balance and why you feel the way you do.

As you work with the elements you will be balancing the chakras associated with them.

More About Doshas
A Brief Overview

KAPHA PEOPLE
Kapha combines the elements of Water and Earth.

A Kapha in balance has tortoise-like stamina as opposed to the flash and burn speed of the hare. Kapha people tend to be more robust and have more physicality than the other Dosha types. A Kapha's temperament will reflect a level-headed approach to life, kindness, generosity, compassion, patience and steadfastness.

The positive qualities we have listed for the root chakra and the Earth element are easy to see in this Dosha personality.

Kapha out of balance or in excess can look like lethargy, insecurity, jealousy, weight gain, hoarding or greedy behavior, even withdrawal from activity. You can see clearly here the relationship to being too heavy in mind, body and spirit, to too much Earth and to a Root chakra that is out of balance.

PITTA PEOPLE
Pitta is a marriage of Fire with some Water. Can you see the steam rising?

Pitta governs metabolism and the integrated processes of the mind, body and spirit. Comprised of two elements that create combustion, Pittas are passionate, intense and intelligent.

A Pitta temperament in balance is organized, ambitious, possesses a lust for life, and makes a natural leader.

An out-of-balance Pitta can err on the side of being competitive and controlling, judgmental and quick to anger.

These are fun, fiery folks. We could all do with some Pitta-style passion. But remember, neither fire nor water is ever still. These are unstable elements that can readily move out of balance and back again. When in balance the elements that make a Pitta tick offer radiant warmth and forward motion.

VATA PEOPLE

The Vata Dosha is composed of the elements of Air and Space. The elements of Air and Space have everything to do with our thoughts and perceptions.

A Vata temperament in balance is quick, clever and highly creative. Vatas love a change of pace and lots of activity, although they may lack in the physical stamina to keep up with their own imagination.

A Vata imbalance can cause worries, insomnia, daydreaming and lack of real productivity.

Too much Vata means being caught in the upper chakra centers and not connecting fully to the physical body. This can result in shyness, insecurity, and lack of stability. The elements of Air and Space are light and easily moved. These are the elements most likely to drift from center - even several times a day under stressful circumstances.

Vatas are like the weather: always changing. Balance here is vital to being present and productive, and enjoying the fun of a well-integrated life.

The nature of the elements and the personalities of the Doshas give us a simple means of recognizing imbalance at its core and an easy entry to chakra balancing. As we take the approach of tapping into the elements as means of coming back to center, our whole yoga practice can be brought in to play.

By combining postures, breathing, compassionate touch and the yoga of lovemaking, you can be lifted up and away from lethargy or wooed back down to earth where your partner awaits you with open arms.

BALANCING YOUR DOSHA
The Art of Re-Centering

Now we will build practice for the most common kinds of imbalance as expressed in the personality traits of the Doshas.

When your Dosha is in balance, you might not even give it a second thought. You feel like you.

We often miss the obvious harmony of being in tune but can quickly identify a "this is not like me" kind of day. To correct the most common kinds of imbalance, you can build a practice that targets the specific personality traits of your Dosha type.

KAPHA OR EARTH/WATER IMBALANCE

When Kapha is out of balance things can get heavy. Kapha contains the essence of the first two chakras, Earth and Water.

These two elements are the densest of the five. The Earth element is the least prone to change. It is usually the last to move out of alignment and the slowest to return.

The root chakra is tied to the Earth element. It is fundamental to our experience of well-being. Getting your foundation steady will support the rest of your life with vitality.

Too much Earth, or a Kapha imbalance, results in lethargy, depression, weight gain or fear of change, as well as feeling dispassionate, withdrawn or stuck in a rut.

To decrease Earth and open a congested root chakra, try the following three postures. As we have mentioned, opposites bring in balance. These postures call on the energies of the upper chakras to draw off excess Kapha or Earth/Water elements.

Use your Basic Yoga Breath throughout.

1. SACRAL ROCKING
The easy fluid movements invite gentle change. The posture moves stagnant energies and births movement from stillness. This is a good place to begin getting unstuck.
2. SPINAL TWIST

From cross legged, turn toward your right. Place your right hand behind you on the floor. Press your palm to the earth and straighten your arm.

Rest your left hand on your right knee. Breathe. Feel warmth moving upward through the length of the spine. Feel the breath like a fluid wave rolling inside your body. Send your awareness to explore your interior space.

Follow the sensation of the inhalation and the exhalation as your whole body expands and contracts with the breath cycle.

Incorporating breath awareness with this posture is detoxifying. It soaks the organs on one side with fresh blood supply while giving the other side a deep cleansing squeeze. Twists rejuvenate the spine and are great for all the glands and organs.

Repeat side to side.

3. CAT STRETCHES
Use the Solo or Partnered variation from Chapters 6 and 7.

Encourage flexibility and motion. Energies begin to flow from the lower chakras upward where they can be assimilated. Energies from the upper chakras flow downward to lighten what was heavy. Use your Ujjayi Breath to make it deeper.

An additional plus: these postures feel good. Even someone who is lethargic will have no difficulty warming up to the three exercises above.

To gently increase your energy level, next move into the following exercises:

4. CAMEL POSE
Use the Solo or Partnered variation from Chapters 6 and 7.

This posture encourages an upward flow of energy. From the firm foundation of the lower body, the upper body awakens. In this pose, the openness of the abdomen, heart, and throat gives rise to the elements of Fire, Air and Space. Hold for several cycles of breath.

5. CAMEL POSE / CHILD'S POSE
Inhale and exhale through the nostrils in slow steady cycles. Hold for six cycles of breath in Camel Pose and then return to Child's Pose for an additional three cycles of breath.

Repeat this Camel to Child's Pose cycle three times. You will notice your energy seem to build and your mind become clear.

To add some heat, try:

6. UPWARD FACING DOG / DOWNWARD FACING DOG
Move with the easy flow of the breath. Allow your breath to carry your body. Move into Up Dog as you inhale and Down Dog as you exhale. This stimulates circulation and oxygen supply to the body and the brain, which will gently cleanse fatigue from your system.

Up Dog primarily stretches the abdomen and chest, making more room for the liver, gall bladder and spleen to function. It also opens the heart and expands the lungs.

Added benefits are a toned butt, a strong flexible back, and shapely legs.

Down Dog releases tension from the whole back body. Your spine extends to its fullest length, which decompresses the discs and opens a steady stream of energy from chakra to chakra. It brings some awareness to the perineum as it is lifted toward the light and gently stretched.

This is great for all the organs and glands.

The practice as a whole will strengthen the body and clear the mind.

Try 5 to 10 rounds of Poses 1 through 6 and then rest in Child's Pose.

Another useful tool to balance your Kapha Dosha, or Earth/Water elements, is massage. A full-body massage, as outlined below, is wonderful. If you need a quicker fix, you can get many benefits from this simple Belly Massage:

Sit at your partner's side. Place your palms warmly on your partner's abdominal area. Move with the relaxed rhythm of your breathing as you lean in toward your partner and then away, creating steady wave-like rocking through the palms of your hands. Cover the whole abdominal area with gentle compressions and releases in a soft kneading action.

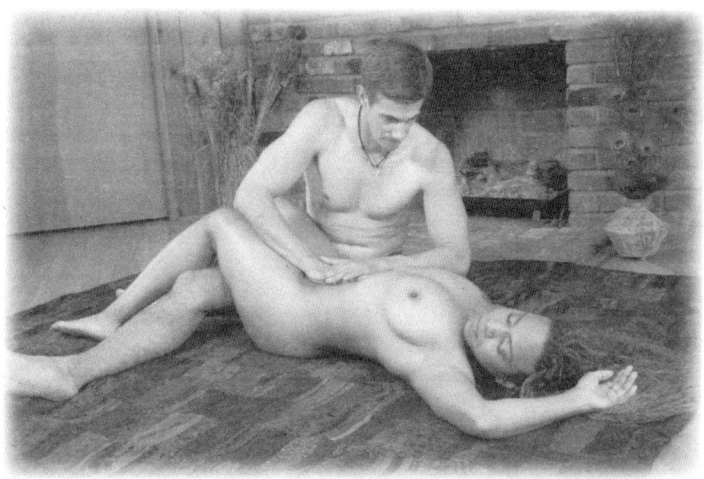

Massage here takes tension from the core of the mind and emotions. It breaks up stagnation in the area of the Sacral chakra and sends a message of freedom and flow to the body/mind.

Full Body Massage
Stretch your partner's arms up and back, making more room to breathe.

The receiving partner should follow the upward-moving sensations in the body: the tingles on the skin... the opening of the abdomen, chest and heart... the enlivening feeling of stretch as gentle heat moving upward through the chest and arms.

Use Sweet Almond oil to lubricate your palms and forearms. Almond is light and won't add excessive oil to Kapha's naturally more oily skin.

Make long gliding upward strokes from the insteps of your partner's feet to their inner thighs.

Now place one hand on the outside and one hand on the inside of your partner's leg. Stroke upward to the top of the thigh.

Repeat with the other leg.

Continue with firm gliding strokes from the hips and buttocks to your partner's heart – both front and back.

Direct your strokes upward with a focus on meeting at the heart center.

Massage the length of each arm. Lift the arms up over the head and massage the hands.

Now use your lightest touch. Tickle your way up toward the heart, breasts, and face. Draw energy right off the top of the head. Give your partner's hair a scalp-stimulating pull. Not too hard – just enough to excite.

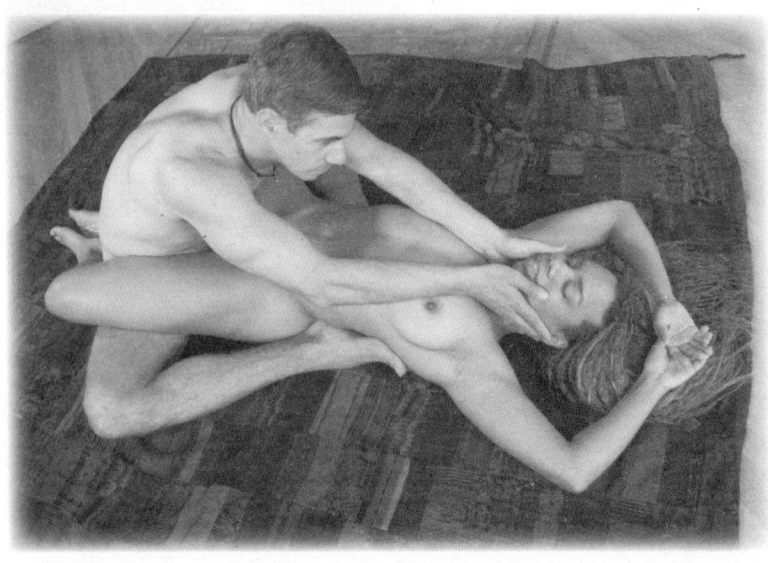

The Yoga of Sex

There are other fun – and sexy – ways that partners can help keep Kapha or Earth/Water elements in balance. The Yoga of Sex is one.

Slow down... celebrate your transition to another level... take time to actually "meet" your partner. Use extended foreplay to warm up. Explore your partner's entire body to find their personal erogenous zones, raising warm tingles and increasing circulation.

A tense, depressed partner needs to relax, making room in the body and mind for ease and freedom. Sex relates to the element of Water, inviting feelings of fluidity to remove a rigid stance in life. The experience of being held and supported encourages letting go. Sexual energies from the 2nd chakra stimulate the release of endorphins to counter depression.

SPOONS - OR LOVER'S FAVORITE POSE
Try Spooning. This sex position is relaxing, intimate and perfect for cuddling before, during, and after sex.

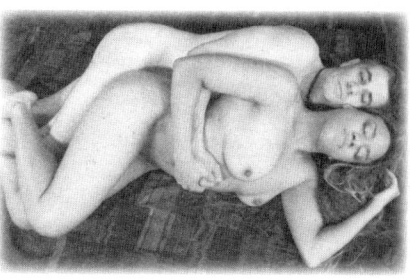

Both partners lie on their sides. The receptive partner presses her back against the active partner's front to rest one inside the other like spoons. The receptive partner parts her legs slightly, with her hips tilted to one side, and her knees bent.

Partners should be positioned so that the penetrative partner's penis is in line with the receptive partner's vagina or anus. With both partners lying on their sides, the man cuddles up into the back of the woman and penetrates her as she draws her knees up toward her stomach.

This position is very intimate and the angle of penetration is great for either G-spot or prostate gland stimulation.

If the woman angles her upper body forward and down toward her partner's feet while her partner does thrusting movements, penetration can be enhanced.

CHILD'S POSE
Child's Pose translates well into a sexual position helpful in balancing Kapha.

From doggy style or on all fours, the receiving partner drops her hips toward her heels, while the active partner moves in close from a kneeling position. His lap makes a soft cushion for the butt and thighs while he pulls her snug to his body.

Child's Pose is a relaxed position to use as a platform for your loving. It is a mild Forward Bend which is soothing. This position can allow the receiving partner to relax her head on a pillow, and exposes the back, butt, and hips to massage while making love.

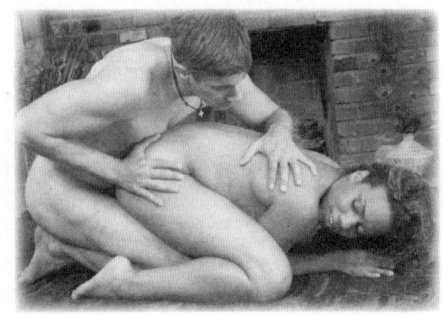

Some people enjoy relinquishing full control to their partner. In this position the active partner controls the depth and speed of penetration. The butt and hips can be lifted up or lowered, making penetration deep or deeper. The active partner also has easy access to the vagina, anus, clitoris and breasts. This position provides excellent G-spot stimulation.

Begin with a soft slow rhythm and steady thrusting. Gradually increase rhythm and speed. Try a combination of shallow thrusts and then deep ones to send stimulating tremors toward the core of her being.

This will break up stagnant Earth energies and invite a lethargic person to experience the joy of movement, shift and the unexpected. As you indulge in the stimulation of Child's Pose, vary your sexual position at least once to bring in movement, change and freedom.

VATA OR AIR/SPACE IMBALANCE
When Vata is imbalanced things can get confusing.

The elements of Space and Air are light and fast moving. Without heavy tethers to the earth, these elements are the most easily thrown off balance during a day due to diet, stress factors, lifestyle, travel and other influences within and beyond your control.

Some common signs of imbalance are constant worry, anxiety, feeling overwhelmed, being tired but too tense to relax, difficulty sleeping, dry skin, chapped lips, feeling spaced out, an inability to focus, and poor memory.

Vatas can become exhausted by their own pace. They need some down time but will resist it.

Physical activity such as yoga will help by moving the activity of a fast mind to the slower pace of the body, one heartbeat at a time.

The complimentary elements of Earth and Water will ease anxiety and invite calm. It's not that we want to tie down a normally light and buoyant type. Rather, we offer tools and touch that provide enough Earth to rest on and the slower pace found in the movement of Water, helping restore equilibrium and soothe frayed nerves.

Yoga Postures
The following postures combine to create a Grounding Yoga Practice, guiding you to meet frenetic mental spin with productive physical activity. Hold the postures a little longer and stronger. This will focus the mind to the single moment of this single activity, easing anxiety and promoting concentration.

Sun Salutations are a good start. Take them at a slow steady pace to encourage grounding through the posture. When you meet each pose, pause for a few cycles of breath and be there and there alone - not already anticipating the next move.

Follow by allowing yourself to hang out in some Forward Bends, inducing relaxation.

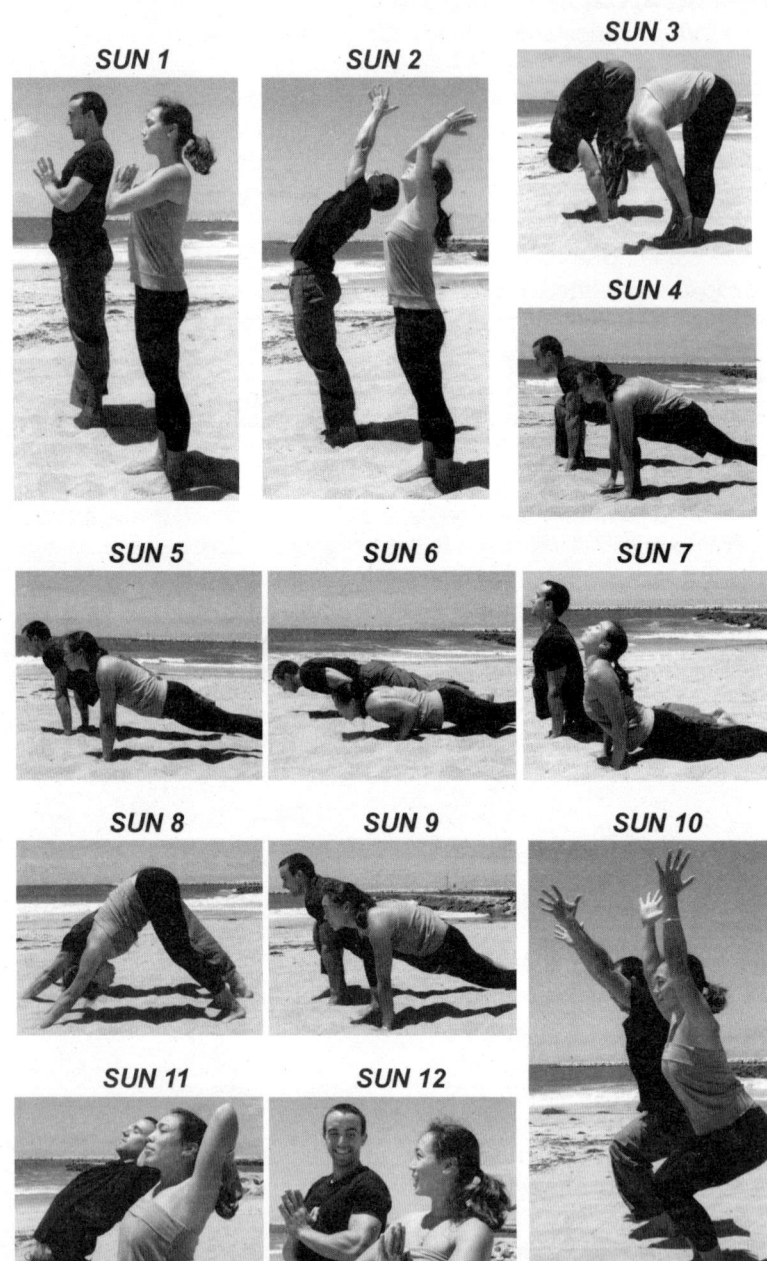

Try **RAGDOLL:**

Plant your feet a hip width apart and hang forward from the hips.

Bend your knees a little for a more relaxed stance.

Let go of the weight of your head, arms, and entire upper body.

Breathe!

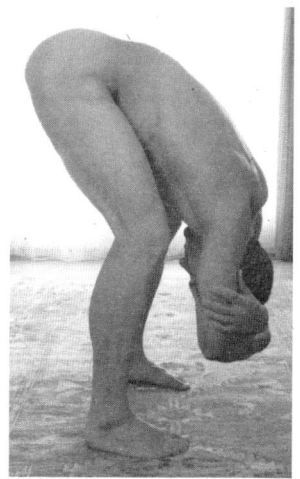

Janu Sirsasana, or Head to Knee Pose, takes you to the floor. It is a stable place to be. Janu Sirsasana relieves tensions from the back, legs, and hips.

Prasarita Padottanasana, or Wide Legged Forward Bend, is great for freeing the back and inducing a more relaxed frame of mind. The feet planted firmly to the floor provide perfect support.

All these poses are explained in detail in Chapter 6 and 7 and all help balance your Vata or Air/Space elements.

CHILD'S POSE
Child's Pose is a universal safe haven for the stressed-out masses that is particularly restorative for an out of balance Vata. It offers the feeling of perfect support, and is grounding and nurturing as your forehead is pillowed on the earth and your body folds comfortably over itself. Gravity is your friend in this pose as it falls through your back and hips, releasing tension. The mind is drawn away from sensory overload and absorbed instead by the calming influence of each breath.

Do this posture alone or savor it as an embrace, using the Partner Yoga variation from Chapter 7. The added feeling of warmth and the present weight of your partner's body offer a dimension of containment and security that translate clearly through the body to the mind. With each exhalation, let your partner's weight settle around you like a warm blanket.

The sedating quality of the breath and the peace inside the posture draw off some of the Space and Air by encouraging what was excess energy to descend through the chakras as a source of nourishment and vitality for the lower chakras.

Breathing Technique
During your yoga practice, inhale slowly through the nostrils and exhale slowly through slightly parted lips. This magnifies the calming qualities available in the Basic Yoga Breath.

Take a moment to simply sit back to back and breathe. The breath itself is a great way to calm down and reenter the present moment by taking the mind out of spin.

Breathing together will increase your feelings of support and interconnectedness.

Massage
Long deep massage strokes are helpful for grounding, and therefore benefit Vata.

Try pure sesame oil for your Vata massage session. It is particularly nourishing for dry skin. Warm your hands by rubbing them briskly together before applying strong gliding strokes that move from your partner's upper body toward her lower extremities.

Use a deep, gliding, pulling movement to work down the length of each arm and leg, including fingers and toes. Add the vibration of gentle shaking to dissipate stress-related tensions. Spend some extra time on her feet, as if willing her down to earth.

Continue your massage by moving to her lower belly and hips. The area just below the navel is our center of gravity, a natural point of balance. Compassionate touch here will deepen the relaxation response and bring up feelings of pleasure. Firmly squeeze, stroke and release the outsides of her hips and the globes of her buttocks several times. When these large muscles get wound up tight they can hinder the fluid movements of the pelvis when making love.

With permission, apply firm palm pressure to the perineum. Try pressing for a full inhalation and relaxing during the exhalation. Breathe together making an "Ahhh" sound as you both exhale.

All of these soothing sensory experiences encourage a downward spiral of energy to calm and contain what was spinning out of control.

The Yoga of Sex

Sex is quite grounding, as it pulls the awareness away from external noise and imbeds it in the pleasure at hand, one soothed nerve at a time. A grounded partner is more emotionally stable, easy-going and calm. The Yoga of Sex is a great way to keep Vata in balance.

These sexual postures encourage relaxation because they give the gift of feeling safe and secure.

FOR HER
Surround her with your body and wrap her inside your arms, your body becoming shelter from the storm. High strung people respond well to gentle physical pressure applied to their body as squeezing and hugging, the same way swaddling calms an infant.

Some of the classic "man on top" positions work best as a calming therapy. Start with just laying together, heart to heart, cheek to cheek, your lower bellies and genitals warmly aligned with or without penetration.

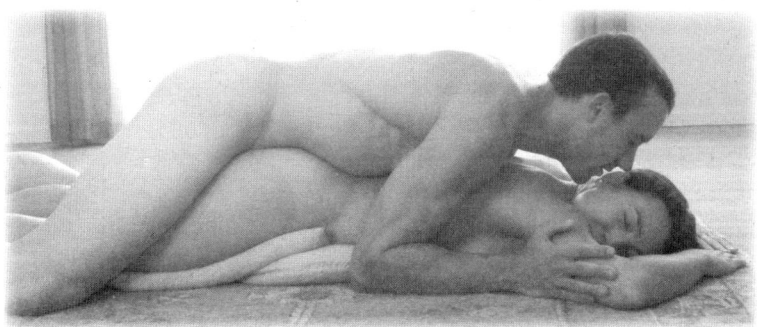

Or turn her face down and rest on top of her back, this position going even further toward complete surrender and passive receiving.

FOR HIM

When your man is in need of grounding sexual therapy, place him in the receptive position. Seating yourself astride his hips, with or without penetration, and leaning forward or back to rest heart to heart is wonderful therapy. As your breathing falls into sync it feels as if you are melting into one another.

Your warm weight, the circle of your arms and the nesting place in between your thighs adds layers of security and contentment as you seem to fill each other.

Try Spooning with him in receptive front position. This is a nice place for you to offer genital massage along with whole body snuggling.

When you are both ready to make love, try rolling face to face in a side-by-side position.

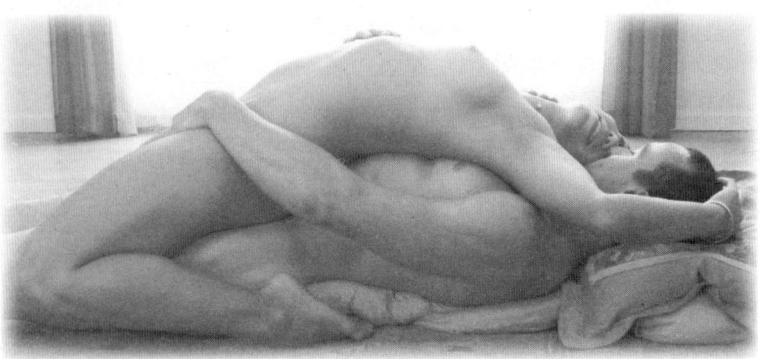

SIDE-BY-SIDE POSITION
Side-by-side as a sexual position is a fine place to start. There is strong eye contact, easy communication, and full access to one another with your curious hands and pleasing fingers. All hands are free to roam the wild terrain of each other's bodies and offer more stimulation to the genitals.

Lie on your sides facing each other. As the man enters the woman with his penis, the woman wraps her leg around her partner's body to facilitate deeper penetration, pulling him toward her with her leg as he thrusts.

Take hold of each other's hips and butt. Encourage strong pelvic movement. Fall into sync, rocking front and back. Feel your pelvis becoming free and fluid.

Let the mind and awareness move into the powerful rhythm of the body. Sighing aloud as you exhale is a powerful means of moving energy in a soothing direction.

Allow the fluidity of the Water element and the security of the Earth element to ground your awareness in the comfort and joy available in the lower chakras. Heavier slower elements of Earth and Water are the natural counter-balance for too much Air and Space. As the imbalance is cleared, your partner will glow with calm strength and enthusiasm and the experience of just being in a body that is having great sex.

When deeper penetration is desired, all it takes is an easy roll over to any variation of man or woman on top postures. *Have fun.*

PITTA OR WATER/FIRE IMBALANCE

When Pitta is imbalanced things can get ugly. The most noticeable traits of excessive Pitta are being irritable and judgmental or exhibiting angry behavior. The unstable elements of Water and Fire are quick to move out of balance. Restoring Pitta to harmony takes a little help from both the upper and lower chakras. All the elements come into play.

Bad mood? Just shake it off by utilizing the Yoga Breath of Joy from Chapter 1. This will meet fire with fire. Some fast vigorous movement will release pent-up frustrations in productive physical activity. Imagine flinging your stress right off the tips of your fingers. Visualize each inhalation as a cooling breeze moving through your overheated engines.

Continue to ground excess energies in an active flow of postures moving at a moderate pace. Try the Sun Salutations as illustrated in the Vata segment above. These postures touch all the primary directions while cleansing the body/mind of tension.

Use Ujjayi breathing throughout this yoga practice for its cooling properties.

Hold each of the following four postures for 5 cycles of breath. Imagine breath coming in through the navel and exiting in all directions, as if through the limbs and the crown of your head, expanding in 5 directions.

Move through:
Warrior One

Warrior Two

Triangle

Forward Bend

Repeat all to the other side.

Move between the next two postures in smooth steady motion. Feel your feet on the ground. Inhale as you lift your hips and exhale as you lower.

EAGLE POSE
A centering balance.
Repeat twice. Hold for as long as 10 cycles of breath.

Into:

SQUAT TO FORWARD BEND
Plant your feet a little wider than your hips. Bend your knees and lower your hips and butt in the direction of your heels. Put each hand palm down on the floor in front of you.

Now inhale, lifting your hips up while folding forward from the waist, lowering your head toward your knees. Exhale, lifting your head while lowering your hips, returning to your initial squat position.

In the following, move with slow fluid grace from posture to posture. Hold each for up to 10 cycles of breath:

BRIDGE POSE...   ***to PLOW POSE...***

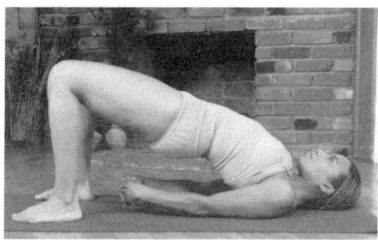 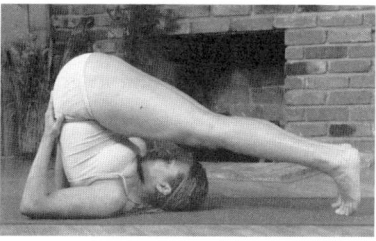

to KNEES TO CHEST POSE...

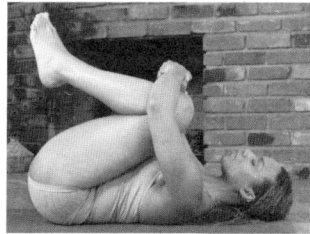

...ending in ***RESTING POSE.***

During your yoga practice you will feel your energies unwind from the top down. The postures work together to engage the mind in the stability and rooted strength of the body.

Warrior One, Warrior Two and Triangle Pose disperse congested energies away from your heated core and outward toward cooling space.

Eagle Pose draws all of your energy and awareness back to a place of rooted vitality.

Squat releases tensions from the hips, which typically hold anger.

The Forward Bend is an invitation to relaxation and further release.

Bridge Pose to Plow Pose eases pent up tensions from the front and back of the spine. They create a full body experience of expanse in Bridge Pose and contract in Plow Pose. The two together bring balance to the body/mind and release stress-related fatigue and irritability.

After resting in Knees to Chest Pose - very relaxing - try:

Alternate Nostril Breathing
Alternate Nostril Breathing brings balance to the physical, emotional and spiritual levels of your being.

To practice, rest your right ring finger on your left nostril and your right thumb on the right nostril.

Close the right nostril and inhale through the left nostril.

Hold the breath a few counts, sealing both nostrils.

Exhale through the right nostril while keeping the left nostril sealed.

Seal both nostrils and hold the breath outside the body for a few counts.

Inhale through the right nostril.

Seal both nostrils for a few counts.

Exhale through the left nostril.

Seal both nostrils and hold the breath outside the body for a few counts.

Continue switching side to side.

Practice for 2-5 minutes. Feel the inner peace.

Massage
As with imbalance in the other two Doshas, a pleasurable way to help regain the Pitta balance you seek is through massage. Try using coconut oil. It's good for a Pitta constitution.

Start with your partner face down. Work down the back with firm gliding strokes from shoulders to buttocks and hips.

Knead the buttocks.

Squeeze and press around the hips.

Work on your partner's feet.

All of this encourages a deeper, calmer state of mind.

When you are ready, turn your partner over for a stimulating Head and Scalp Massage. This feels so wonderful it can even relieve a headache.

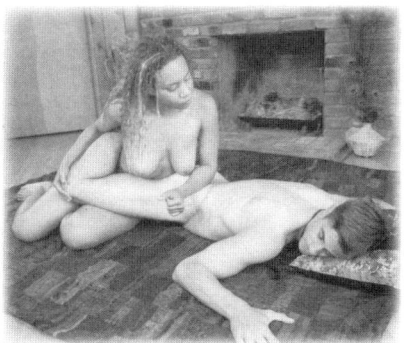 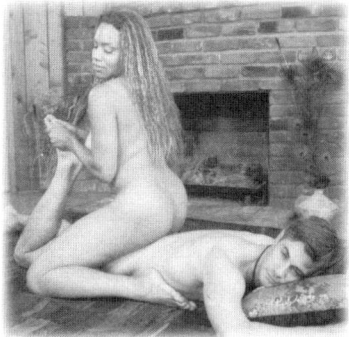

Jaw Massage is an addition your partner will thank you for. It helps release tensions we sometimes don't even realize we have - those accumulated from clenching the jaw and teeth in those stress-filled moments that occur throughout the day.

A Belly Massage disperses tension from the core and brings the whole being back into balance. It's a quick, easy way to pamper a Pitta or Water/Fire element that is unbalanced.

If you'd like to try the following full-body technique for a Belly Massage, you may enjoy being the giver as much as your partner enjoys receiving it.

Roll on top of your partner and apply long, sensual, full-body strokes.

Press your chest to their low abdomen and glide upward to their chest and back again. Feel the friction making sparks of pleasure everywhere you touch.

The Yoga of Sex

Passion is Pitta's forte. Work out any imbalance by trying sex positions that offer easy movement for both of you. The therapy here is all about pace. Slow down. Follow the sensations in your touch. How slowly can you enter your partner? How completely can you follow the excitement your nerve endings are sending back to command central? Let anticipation cast a deeper spell. Build up slowly and extend your pleasure.

Don't settle for a cheap thrill when you can enjoy a long satisfying exchange. You will both feel relaxed and renewed.

FOR HER
Try a Man on Top position to refresh Pitta's energy.

Go ahead and give him permission to pleasure you. From his perch on top he can easily manipulate her pelvis to roll front and back or rock her hips side to side while resting his weight between her thighs, penetrating deeply.

She can relax and enjoy his ability to pleasure her breasts and clitoris, or enjoy stimulating them herself to maximize the pleasures at hand.

Though she seemingly relinquishes control, she can be active and able to respond with pelvic thrusting and rocking.

A change of pace is as simple as pulling her knees toward her chest for deeper penetration or twisting her hips to one side, changing the angle of his thrusting and finding new areas inside the vagina to stimulate.

Some women get better G-spot massage from the penis with this kind of twisting and rolling exchange.

Or try:

TIGER TAO

This rear entry position allows for deep penetration and vigorous thrusting rather than tender lovemaking. The woman positions herself on all fours as in Cat Stretches, with her man kneeling behind her.

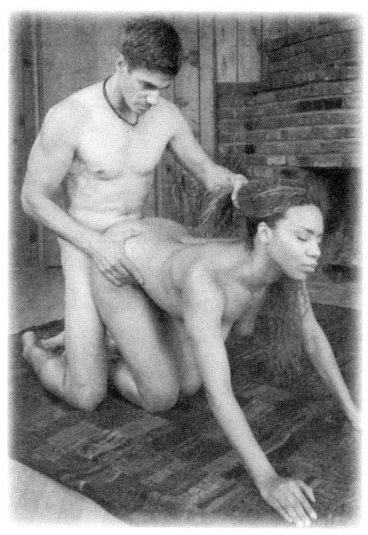

Both partners are active, though he is in control of the depth and speed of the encounter. She can flex and round her back to change the angle of his penis as it slides in and out. He can hold onto her hair, sensually taking command of her body, or hold onto her shoulders for more support.

From here he can hit the G-spot easily and move up against the cervix if it feels good to her. Cervical stimulation creates waves of vibration that sometimes resonate to the core, resulting in small uterine contractions - which in this case feel insanely good.

This position also allows the man to caress his partner's breasts, buttocks and clitoris.

FOR HIM
Try Woman on Top positions for a male Pitta who needs some nurture.

In the WOMAN ON TOP / ASTRIDE POSITION:
The man lies on his back and the woman sexily lowers herself onto his erect penis.

Facing him, she may squat with both feet planted to either side of his body. Or kneel, supporting herself with her hands on his chest, shoulders or the bed.

Bending forward, she can massage his chest, tweak his nipples or kiss his face, ears and neck.

In this position, she is in control of the speed and the depth of penetration. She can vary the angle of his penis inside her vagina.

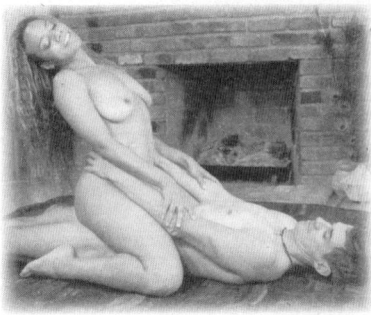

Leaning her upper body forward results in more G-spot stimulation. Leaning backward, supporting her back with her hands behind her, results in more direct deep thrusts and incredible pleasure for both. It presents a very sexy view of both her body taking him in and her growing arousal.

Sitting on top, she can also turn, facing away from him and looking in the direction of his feet. This "Reverse Cowgirl" position once again changes the depth and area of stimulation for her while he enjoys both the view and her excitement.

With her in control, he can lay back and receive, moving all of his awareness into his body. As excitement leads to orgasm, he can delight in letting go and being out of control.

After the lovemaking reaches its climax, the Rx here is to stay connected. Allow the soft penis to rest inside her vagina.

Breathe together and continue to move into a place of expanse. Follow all the tendrils of energy where they lead you. Allow the mind and emotions to flow along with all of the tingly sensations in the body.

Let go of tension in your jaw, brow, butt and genitals. Let feelings of peace and pleasure expand through your body and mind.

Enjoy feeling alive and resonant with glowing balanced energy that wraps both of you up in its arms.

In closing...

Yoga means many things to many people.

Yoga translates as union. That union extends from a union of one's self to the soul and beyond, one's self to the mind, body and emotions, and most delightfully to one's self in joyous union with another.

You can benefit from any of these mind body techniques as they best suit your mood, time, and situation. Our aim here is to use the very same stressors that usually cause couples to quarrel to create instead a fun, sensual, sexual healing.

Who needs "make-up sex" when you can avoid the fight and instead stay present to the love you share.

This mode of approach invites deeper intimacy, better communication, and sizzling sex.

Enjoy!

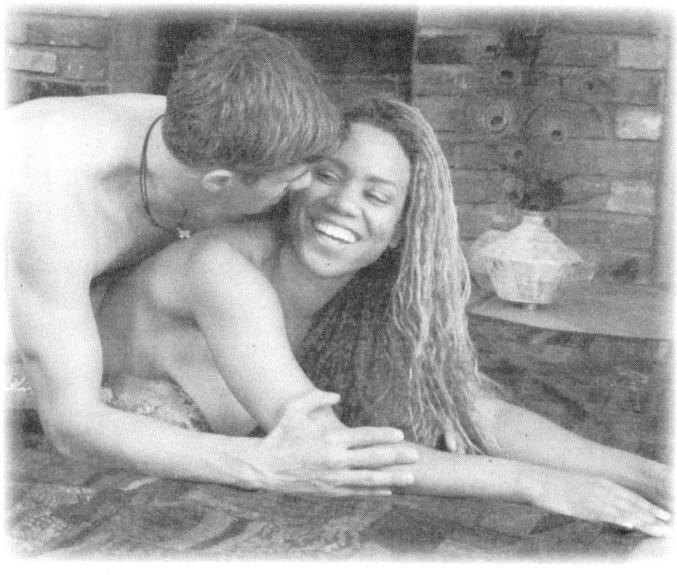

Chapter 10: Sex as Good Medicine
The Healing Power of Pleasure

The latest buzz about sex tells us that "abstinence should only be practiced in moderation."

A safe and healthy sex life should be considered a magic bullet that inoculates not only against loneliness but improves the quality of your life and the quantity of its days. Recent studies show that sex plays a vital role in heart health, brain function and psychological well-being.

Finally... something that feels this good really is good for you!

If you need encouragement to rev up your sex life read on.

The life affirming joys of sex in an intimate relationship can become a potent source of healing and renewal.

Tension is released during orgasm, leaving the whole body/mind system purring with vitality. Pleasure invites deep relaxation, a condition of openness and receptivity that can elevate your consciousness by opening a window to the bliss nature of the soul.

Recent studies clearly show that a healthy sex life is about much more than procreation and recreation. Sex is tied directly to our vitality in a number of ways.

When we enjoy mutually caring sexual intimacy, the endocrine system releases a magic potion of neurochemicals and hormones that pour through the body/mind.

It is this elixir of life that blesses us with that in love feeling and is the now recognized as the new miracle drug for overall well-being.

Did you know that orgasms stimulate and increase the secretions of the pineal and pituitary glands? This affects brain chemistry by fueling the endocrine glands with more hGH, serotonin, DHEA, and testosterone, strengthening not only the endocrine system but the immune and nervous functions, leading to improved sexual health, rejuvenation and longevity.

hGH, or human Growth Hormone, assists in the battle against aging. Reported effects include decreased body fat, increased muscle mass, increased bone density, increased energy levels, improved skin tone and texture, and improved immune system function.

Serotonin plays an important role in the central nervous system as a neuro-transmitter in the modulation of anger, aggression, body temperature, mood, sleep, human sexuality, appetite, and metabolism.

DHEA, produced by adrenal glands, has been called the "mother of all hormones." Some claim it can help us live longer, lose weight or gain it, prevent cancer, heart disease, and Alzheimer's and combat AIDS and other infectious diseases.

Testosterone plays a key role in health and well-being, as well as in osteoporosis, in men. On average, an adult human male body produces about forty to sixty times more testosterone than an adult female body, but females are, from a behavioral perspective, more sensitive to the hormone.

The power of sexual pleasure can lift depression, lighten migraines, diminish physical pain, support your cardiovascular system, sharpen your senses and stabilize your emotions. Frequent sex works the muscles of the pelvic floor, easing PMS, reversing incontinence and clearing urinary tract issues in women. Spinal flexibility, so important to maintaining youthfulness and assuring longevity, is encouraged and even gained through the playful dance of your hips during sex. Every wave of pleasure ignites a similar freedom of movement in the body while promoting the flow of vital spinal fluids.

More? Your playful romp in between or on top of the sheets is a powerful anti-ageing treatment, making your eyes sparkle and years fall off of your face as the effects of stress are wiped away with that post coital glow.

Frequent and powerful orgasms increase the level of the orgasm hormone, oxytocin. Your oxytocin level is linked to the personality, passion, social skills and emotional quotient (EQ), all of which affects career, marriage, emotions and social life. Orgasms are potent elixirs that encourage more sexual health because they empower our pituitary (brain function.)

Of course sex is an opportunity for a much deeper union than just a basic genital connection of pronged point A into circuit connection B. More sex by itself is not the whole prescription. Emotional intimacy and spiritual connection is a large part of sexual completeness and lasting satisfaction. This is where your Partner Yoga practice comes into play!

The close contact, deep relaxation and nurturing touch found in your partnered practice will also flood your system with endorphins. Intimacy on this more subtle scale can fill the gaps between sex and those occasional dry spells between relationships.

In short : All pleasurable experiences that satisfy a need for human touch go a long way toward making a whole, happy you.

It is here again that the raw force of our sheer physiological energy is treated to the refining touch of the Chakras. We are a body, a mind, emotions, and an indomitable spirit. These aspects of self rub up against each other in a constant interweaving of matter and spirit that span the dimensions. There are no gaps. We are all that.

In understanding both the physical component of each Chakra as it relatesto the endocrine system and the emotional aspects of your being that are influenced by these energy centers, you have an opportunity to choose to create an exceptional sex life and an enlightened state of mind.

Your Partner Yoga practice as a whole can bring about the same kind of hormonal balance and rejuvenation as conscious touch, full presence, full body contact, and a deeply relaxed and receptive state of mind flood your endocrine system with fresh energies.

Chapter 11: The Art of After
A Few Thoughts to Follow Lovemaking

Follow the afterglow and see where it goes.

We often expect sex to give us the loving emotional connection we crave with our partner. We often think that sex will fulfill every need. We are often let down and left disillusioned.

The practice you have learned will go a long way toward making your sex life something to shout about while showing you the way to fulfilling the cry of your heart for a deeper connection – a true sense of oneness that is about far more than sexual satisfaction alone.

Our partnered practice of yoga prepared the body, heart and mind for the deeper union of sex.

Sexual union with your beloved lover now prepares you to experience even greater feelings of intimacy through using your naturally sensual being to access unmet places in the spirit.

Rather than roll over and go to sleep or jump up to do something else, take advantage of all the beautiful energies you have opened up during lovemaking to explore the unseen dimensions where the two of you have virtually become one.

Every good yoga session should be followed by resting in Savasana or "corpse pose." Savasana allows time for the energies kindled during the physical practice of yoga to meld, creating a state of true balance that is unique to you and you alone. Our practice has been geared to support sexual fabulousness and emotional harmony. This resting place is a chance to extend the feelings of connection found in the body to reach toward the union of heart and soul.

So after all the physical energy is spent, rest together in simple sweet embrace.

~ Follow the afterglow and see where it goes ~

How? We will simply consider a few questions...

What does your body feel like right after orgasmic sex?

Start with the deep pulsing reverberations echoing from your sexual core.

Feel, listen, and reach into the sensations you feel there.

Allow feelings of pleasure to expand...

Touching body, mind, and soul as one.

Where is there heat in your body?

Where does it go?

Tap into the part of you that is light and energy.
Follow the heat in your body as it moves through your skin to fill the space around you.
Glow.

Where does Love live in your body?

Find it.
Follow it.
Fan its gentle flame into every cell.
Expand your sense of self toward your partner.

Where do you seem to touch, overlap, mingle and sing?

Breathe into the micro spaces between you until all is one thing.
Send the breath back and forth between you.
Move into subtle ebb and flow, each breath knitting you together.

Inhale love.
Exhale love.

Where does space become connection?
Where do you start and end?

Is there an end?

Be like two rivers merging, flowing as one into a greater open sea.
Be the sea.
Be the light dancing on the waters.
Be the smile on the face of your lover.
Be the heart and its beat.

Rest together as if this is the only moment in the Universe.
Be the Universe and know the limitlessness of a moment.

How is this miracle possible?

Extend your most heartfelt Namaste to one another.

~ *Namaste* ~

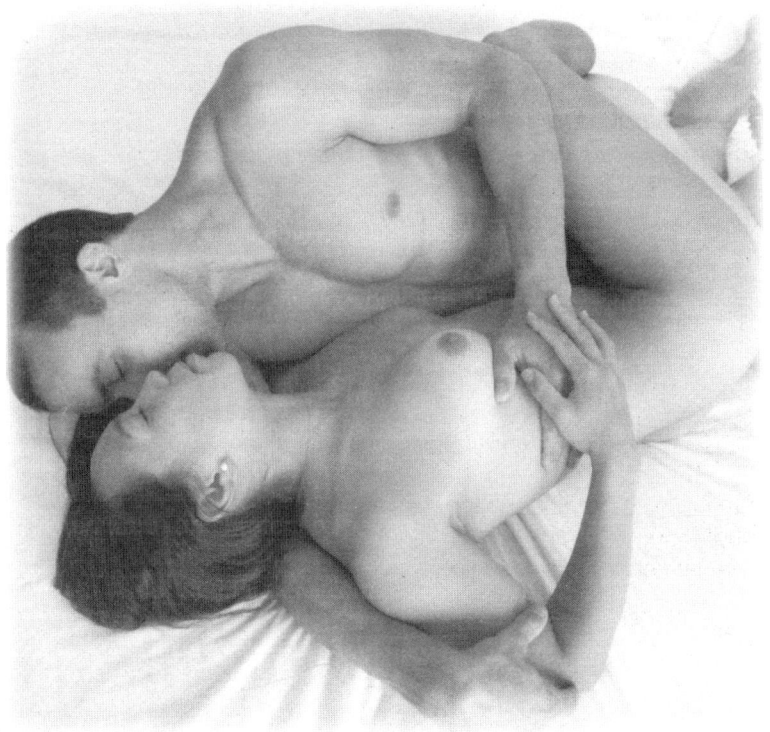

An exclusive offer for readers of this book:

70% OFF
your entire first order of
streaming videos from Loving Sex,
the world's largest
tastefully explicit sex education series

Visit **www.aivid.net**

Use the code **PC2470** during checkout

Real couples. Real Sex. Real Life.

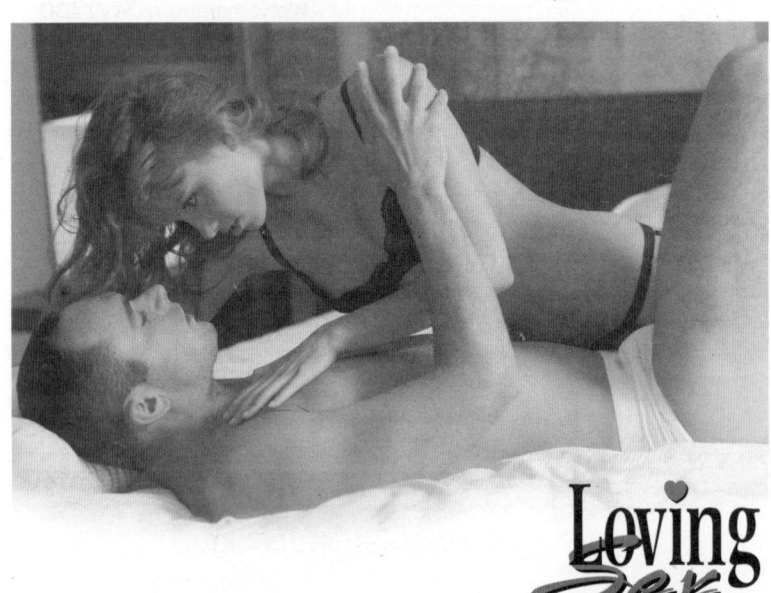